THE USE AND ABUSE
OF MEDICINE

THE USE AND ABUSE OF MEDICINE

Edited by
Marten W. de Vries
Robert L. Berg
Mack Lipkin, Jr.

PRAEGER

PRAEGER SPECIAL STUDIES • PRAEGER SCIENTIFIC

Library of Congress Cataloging in Publication Data
Main entry under title:

The Use and abuse of medicine.

Bibliography: p.
Includes index.
1. Social medicine—Addresses, essays, lectures.
2. Medical anthropology — Addresses, essays,
lectures. 3. Medical care—Addresses, essays, lectures. I. de Vries, Marten W. II. Berg, Robert L.
III. Lipkin, Jr., Mack. [DNLM: 1. Attitude to health.
2. Cross-cultural comparisons. 3. Medicine.
4. Sociology, Medical. WA 30 U84]
RA418.U75   362.1   82-7563
ISBN 0-03-061702-2   AACR2

Published in 1982 by Praeger Publishers
CBS Educational and Professional Publishing
a Division of CBS, Inc.
521 Fifth Avenue, New York, New York 10175, U.S.A.

© 1982 by Praeger Publishers

23456789   145   987654321

Printed in the United States of America

CONTENTS

PART IV: TOO MUCH OR TOO LITTLE MEDICALIZATION

PART V: THE INTERFACE BETWEEN WESTERN AND
        TRADITIONAL MEDICINE

vii

PART VI: ON THE USE AND ABUSE OF MEDICINE: A CONCLUSION
Marten W. de Vries, Robert L. Berg, and Mack Lipkin, Jr.

FOREWORD

The 1970s began at the peak of an era of high funding, the war on cancer was an analogy to the space race, and intense optimism existed about the molecular biological revolution and the potential of biotechnical approaches to medical care. Then came a series of critiques that presented medicine less as miracle than as monster. The most visible of these, Illich's *Medical Nemesis: The Expropriation of Health* presented a view of medicine as more harmful than helpful, as creating more disease and dependency than its treatments cured. Medicine was part of the problem rather than a system of solutions. Similarly, Carlson, in *The End of Medicine*, prophesied that the Flexnerian medical system, built in the United States since 1912 and typified by such institutions as Harvard, Johns Hopkins, and the National Institutes of Health, had become irrelevant to the health of the public, dangerous to people with common problems, and outmoded and nasty in how it dealt with people. On a more scholarly and less rhetorical plane, McKeown, in *The Role of Medicine: Dream, Mirage or Nemesis*, declared that the role of medicine in the twentieth century has become primarily that of prevention and comfort and that medicine has little effect on the health of populations.

Those of us in the actual practice of medicine, burdened with humanistic concerns and interested in analytical approaches to caring for people, felt troubled by these critiques. Certainly many of the examples were valid and telling. Yet it seemed that the criticisms of Illich, Carlson, McKeown, Szasz, and others often denied the basic human necessity that there be medicine and overlooked what seemed to be the sincerity and strenuousness of effort of some practitioners to understand how to be truly helpful. The criticisms seemed overblown, overgeneralized, and unconstructive.

The jargon phrase used by these critics is that there is too much "medicalization." This means that medicine has spread too broadly into areas that do not concern it. It has overstepped its domain and become too dominant an aspect of social life. This perspective influenced both health care policy makers and the citizenry, and medicine was subjected to increased regulation. Although the critique sounded reasonable enough, the basic premise passed unanalyzed. The overmedicalization critique seemed particularly off the mark to those of us who had studied traditional societies in which the integration of health care with community life was viewed as a positive value to be emulated in the West. Contradictions of this sort motivated the clinicians, ethnographers, and historians who write here to examine the medicalization critique more closely.

The contributors to this book seek not to address or redress the sorts of critiques described above but to find their proper context. They examine, through several interdisciplinary lenses, the issue of the proper place of medicine. First, a theoretical approach is undertaken by anthropologists, medical theorists, and a historian. Then a specific illness entity, couvade, is examined cross-culturally in considerable detail and analyzed from sociological and medical-theoretical points of view. Finally, a variety of case studies from multiple disciplines and settings, ranging from the West to the Third World enrich the data points from which to create a picture of the proper place of medicine.

The novel response to the critique provided in this book is that the critique itself is too narrow. While the specific criticisms are often correct, the notion that this is because medicine is becoming too broad and invasive is less correct than that medicine fails to know when and how to be *appropriate*. This volume evolves this view through a rich cross-cultural, historical, and medical matrix of articles.

This book grew out of a conference in Rochester, New York, supported by the University of Rochester's Rochester Plan and sponsored by the Departments of Preventive, Family, and Rehabilitation Medicine, Psychiatry, and Anthropology. The volume, however, is not merely a conference proceedings. Articles in addition to those presented at the conference were solicited to round out the arguments. Much cross referencing has taken place. Less germane papers, while excellent, were not included. At our direction most of the papers underwent major revision. We have been helped in this by the Rochester Plan and by the Rockefeller Foundation. As well, we acknowledge the assistance of many friends and colleagues. We thank all who have helped in the editing and writing of this work as well

as our editor, Jerry L. Stone of Praeger, who has graciously facilitated the excellent production of this book.

Marten W. de Vries
Cambridge, Massachusetts

Robert L. Berg
Rochester, New York

Mack Lipkin, Jr.
New York, New York
1982

INTRODUCTION:
MEDICALIZATION IN PERSPECTIVE

Marten W. de Vries

Under the halo of the germ theory, medicine grew encouraged by the hopes of humanity that it would eradicate most diseases. Medical approaches, particularly over the past 30 years, have spread into the community and family as preventive programs, and prescribed health ways for social intercourse became part of daily life. During this period the doctor-patient relationship extended beyond treatment when illness strikes to self-care education, including encouraging constructive attitudes toward exercise, diet, blood pressure, cigarette smoking, and the management of stress at home and work.

With this growth of medicine and the related biomedical research establishment, the perception grew that the benefits of new medical approaches were not equally distributed to the population. Various efforts, such as neighborhood health center programs and medicaid and medicare programs were created to adjust its most obvious shortcomings. As a result, medical and health-related activities came to increasing public attention. People began not to take their health care system lightly. Articles defining health, decrying cost, and demystifying medical care appeared regularly in the lay and professional literature. Today, the belief that science-based medicine would be a triumphant procession is in doubt. Instead, medicine is criticized for contributing to an array of social, financial, and medical problems.

The questions of how much and what kind of medicine is genuinely required for social and personal well-being and at what cost this should be achieved have become dominant social concerns. While utopian aspirations for health are held by both practitioner and citizen alike, medical care is often experienced by the patient as remote and dehumanizing and by other professionals as competitive for limited medical resources (Unschuld, 1975). The conflict between health expectations and the limitations of medical care have led to a skeptical view about medical activities and its unplanned expansion. Medicine has attempted self-healing adjustments, such as peer review systems, self-care education for patients, and the rendering of community services. These well-meaning changes have often led to the further institutionalization of medical approaches without clear benefit. Has medicine therefore become a giant that has overstepped its domain, interfering with the therapeutic functions of other social units such as the family, the community, and the self-healing capacity of the individual (Illich, 1976)?

Medicine is criticized as having overmedicalized society (Illich, 1976; Carlson, 1975; Szasz, 1961). A praiseworthy aim of these critics is to decrease physician-caused ills, i.e., iatrogenesis. Illich (1976), the most visible proponent of this point of view, discusses three levels of iatrogenesis that render medicine a "nemesis": (1) production of pain, sickness, and death at the clinical level; (2) reinforcement of industrial ill health at the social level; and (3) reduction of autonomous self-healing behavior and the healing potential of other social networks at the cultural level. This criticism is an attack on professional dominance and not primarily a complaint about the dominance of ideas about health (Fox, 1977). The critique of professional dominance comes from both the political left and right (Navarro, 1976) and is evidenced in the general population by the numerous health care alternatives that flourish today. In the medicalization critique, biomedicine is viewed as abusive in that it is (1) an authoritarian class and culture-bound orientation that creates dependency and limits individual freedom under the guise of securing ideal health (Illich, 1976); (2) a competitor for limited world resources (Unschuld, 1979); or (3) merely a pawn, a repository of values defined by more powerful interests in the international system (Navarro, 1975).

Medicine's critics find their mark in what they view as irrational conspiratorial and self-aggrandizing medical activity. These allegations have led health planners and skeptics alike to reevaluate the nature of medical care in the West. What remains unclear, however, is whether the medical profession has been successful in creating dependency. If this is the case, are the reasons to be found in the general population that make it more compliant and receptive to professional dominance or in the imperial success of the professions in persuading a reluctant public?

The medicalization critics clearly assign culpability to medicine's more questionable motives. From another perspective, however, the power and evolution of the medical profession is contingent on the approval and support of a wider public. Support for medical activities may wax and wane independent of efforts by the profession. Medicine is deeply embedded in the social system (Stevens, 1971; Foucault, 1973). A clear understanding of the context of medical activity is then required to make sense of the medicalization critique.

In this volume we identify medical and social issues that have led to the encroachment of medicine into modern life and offer an evaluation of medical activity and expansion in historical and cultural perspective. Three approaches are used: (1) a comparative look at medical systems active in different societies today, (2) an analysis of a specific illness in two cultures (New Guinea and New York), and (3) a historical and observational analysis of Western medical activity on location in the West and in the Third World.

DYNAMICS OF MEDICAL SYSTEM AND MEDICALIZATION

Therapeutic activities are highly visible elements of every society. They are important, if not crucial, statements about the relationship between humanity, society, and environment. Until the recent growth of the subdiscipline of medical anthropology, simplistic perspectives prevailed about the relationship of non-Western societies to health and disease. These ranged from a condescending view of a fatalistic, sickly, and backward people huddled in fear from their dimly understood universe to a romantic picture of preindustrial life as psychologically and physically harmonious with the environment. Today, cross-cultural studies in medicine have opened our eyes to the great variation in human adaptive responses to the environment and have highlighted the variation in medical systems across groups that vary in race, culture, and geography.

From these studies the medical or health care system emerged as a subsystem among other systems in society. The notion of medical activity as a system is heuristically useful to us in clarifying the issue of medicalization and conceptualizing alternative approaches in medical care.

Medical systems are delicately interwoven with a group's ideas and feelings about physical events and the range of its social activities. They play a crucial role in classifying emotional and physical states into illness categories (Fabrega, 1974). They are a guardian and repository for the classification of physical and social events (Navarro, 1975).

Ethnographic and historical data suggest that medical systems, to the extent that they are identifiable institutions, vary from culture to culture in concert with social, physical, and historical factors (Alland, 1970; Kleinman, 1980). Historically, medical systems rise, come to power, may be challenged, and fall (Janzen, 1982). They may act as corporate entities (Fortes, 1969), being loose bags of therapeutic activities that exist only in sporadically organized, one-to-one group exchanges (Katz, 1981). Politically, they may act as conservative instruments policing sociocultural properties (Illich, 1976) or may be reactive, often radical elements facilitating growth and change (Elling, 1978). The evolution of the role and characteristics of the medical system seems linked to the degree of differentiation and complexity of the social group. The degree of its autonomy from other systems increases with the degree of specialization and technological sophistication (Fabrega, 1974).

In modern industrial societies, medical activity has shifted from the family to a professionalized, established medical system (Illich, 1976), diminishing the integrated relationship of the medical system with the totality of social life. In the setting in which medicine is ethically and geographically removed from the face-to-face controls of community life, the notion of restricting medical power evolved. In the absence of these controls, medical activity grows suspect, seemingly having the potential to lead us into an oppressive therapeutic society, justified by the medical model, reinforced by coercive labeling (Brown, 1976), and policed by health-related community services (Kunitz, 1974).

Modern medicine is a double-edged sword. While improving health, it may gain for itself and its guardians increased economic and social control. By expanding its involvement in society, it may bleed the strength of social healing networks. Furthermore, its role in improving health remains debatable since there is evidence that biomedicine has not had as positive an influence on world health as has been ascribed to it. Most of the major epidemiological shifts for which modern medicine takes some credit are the primary result of other forces, such as sanitation and decreased crowding (McKeown, 1976; McNeil, 1976).

In the United States, medical activity crossed the threshold to public awareness as medical expenses approached 10 percent of the gross national product and became a major economic factor in society (Richmond, 1981). The complex critiques of medicine seek to diminish professional medicine's ability to allocate resources to itself. Medical criticism then represents in part a political struggle for resource reallocation. Medicine has undoubtedly grown opportunistically since World War II, yet while competitive it has also been co-opted by other social and industrial interests. It has been vulnerable to external control (Navarro, 1975) and abuse as a political tool. This is exemplified by George Vincent, who stated in 1916 that "for the purpose of placating primitive people medicine has some advantages over machine guns" (Brown, 1976).

In the West, as the acknowledged domain of medicine extended into areas that had previously not been considered part of medicine, medicalization occurred. If medicalization is a process with constructive analytical utility, should it not be identifiable within the health care system of traditional cultures as well as the West? An inquiry into the medical system in traditional cultures, however, points to a contradiction between the medicalization critique and data supplied by ethnographical studies of other cultures. In these studies, traditional medical systems often demonstrate an integrated relationship with the rest of society. The medicalization criticism, however, criticizes precisely this integration of activities in the Western system, that is, the increased involvement of modern medicine in day-to-day life.

Medical systems, created to battle illnesses for the social group, do so with complicated and varied consequences. Health, the coveted outcome, remains an ideal concept, difficult to define or measure. The World Health Organization's definition of health as the total physical, mental, and social well-being of an individual is more a striving than a state people can achieve. The authors in this volume tend to view health and illness as complexly caused and interrelated with other aspects of life. The experience and conceptualization of health and illness are viewed as closely linked to the health care system (Kleinman, 1980; Lipkin and Kupka, 1982). A medical system's adequacy is the context-dependent well-being and health of its people. The feeling of well-being, however, is a complexly determined individual state. It should not be simply equated with medical activities. We caution that health is not what doctors do. What doctors do, depends on how well they do it, and what they should perhaps do better is one aspect of the sociocultural perspective on the medicalization critique that we shall pursue further in this book, while expanding our models and perspectives on clinical care.

THE USES AND ABUSES OF MEDICINE

In Part I, the forces that mold, maintain, and motivate medical systems are examined. Historical and comparative cases are used to clarify the interplay of a group's level of development, its available technology, and its illness taxonomy. Conclusions about medicalization are drawn from observed medical activity in a variety of settings. Medicalization is viewed as a systematic principle of medical systems that must be reckoned with by the clinical and social scientist alike, as a process inseparable from general socialization in a culture, and as a process vulnerable to factors such as available resources, technology, and manpower.

In Part II "becoming an illness" uses couvade, the experience of pregnancy-related symptoms by the mates of expectant women, as the analytic focus. Here, symptoms derived in a specific life cycle setting are analyzed through an in-depth comparison of two cultures. The interaction of culture, symptom formation, and the nature of the health system are examined in detail and produce an answer to the medicalization critique. In the previous chapters, medical systems were viewed as functioning by means of a taxonomy of health and disease. The illness taxonomy defines what is medical. The expansion of this taxonomic control through the labeling of human experience is a prime instrument of medicalization. The discussion of couvade highlights this labeling process by contrasting the relatively narrow taxonomy and view of illness in the Western medical system to the complex interactions and integrated relationships of couvade phenomena with social life in a small New Guinea tribe. The differences clarify the large number of factors actually necessary for a full understanding of an illness process.

Part III discusses how cultures organize around the fact of illness. Focus is on the evaluation of the appropriateness of the paradigms used to guide clinical care. Diverse approaches to health care are illustrated both within and without orthodox medical systems. The discussion focuses on the role of resources in regulating medical activity, the multiple and hierarchical strategies of patients throughout the world, and socialization and training processes influencing medical care in the West.

Part IV examines how much and what kinds of medicine are helpful. A historical example from Bismarckian Germany highlights the *rhetorical* abuse of medical approaches. An analysis of current health care provisions for the chronically ill who are not adequately tended to in America is offered as an exmple of "too little" medicalization. "Too little" and perhaps the "wrong kind" of medicine are discussed, concerning infectious disease eradication projects in African populations with leprosy. This example stresses again the need for more comprehensive and informed medical care.

Part V examines the interface of biomedicine with traditional medicine in developing countries. While Western medical activities have improved the well-being of many people, traditional healing methods have often been inappropriately neglected. Inadvertently, or with mixed motivations, the expansion of Western medicine has had negative consequences along with positive gains. The discussion underscores the risk of undermining traditional medical approaches and the care required in international medical activity to extract the best from both models. This is difficult, given the seductive links of modern medicine with other modernizing forces in the Third World and the intolerance of Western medicine for its less "scientific" cousins.

Part VI synthesizes the points of view derived from comparative and historical frameworks presented in the volume. The conclusion calls for health care efforts that fit people's lives in context.

REFERENCES

Alland, A. 1970. *Adaptation in Cultural Evolution: An Approach to Medical Anthropology*. New York: Columbia.
Brown, E. 1979. *Rockefeller Medicine Men*. Berkeley: University of California Press.

Carlson, R. 1975. *The End of Medicine*. New York: Wiley-Interscience.

Elling, R. H. 1978. Medical Systems as Changing Social Systems. *Soc. Sci. Med.* 12:197-215.

Fabrega, H. 1974. *Disease and Social Behavior: An Interdisciplinary Perspective.* Cambridge, Mass.: M.I.T. Press.

Fortes, M. 1969. *Kinship and the Social Order*. Chicago: Aldine.

Foucault, M. 1973. *Birth of the Clinic: An Archeology of Medical Perception.* New York: Random House.

Fox, R. 1977. The Medicalization and Demedicalization of American Society. In *Doing Better and Feeling Worse*, ed. J. Knowles. New York: Norton.

Illich, I. 1976. *Medical Nemesis: The Expropriation of Health*. New York: Pantheon.

Janzen, J. M. 1982. *Lemba 1650-1930, A Drum of Affliction in Africa and the New World*. New York: Garland.

Katz, R. 1981. Education as Transformation: Becoming a Healer among the !Kung and the Fijians. *Harvard Educ. Rev.* 51(11).

Kleinman, A. 1980. *Patients and Healers in the Context of Culture*. Berkeley: University of California Press.

Kunitz, S. 1974. Professionalism and Social Control in the Progressive Era: The Case of Flexner Report. *J. Soc. Problems* 22:16-27.

Lipkin, M. and K. Kupka. 1982. *Psychosocial Problems Affecting Health*. New York: Praeger.

McKeown, T. 1976. *The Role of Medicine: Dream, Mirage or Nemesis*. Princeton, N.J.: Princeton University Press.

McNeil, W. H. 1976. *Plagues and Peoples*. New York: Anchor Press/Doubleday.

Navarro, V. 1975. The Industrialization of Fetishism or the Fetishism of Industrialism: A Critique of Ivan Illich. *Soc. Sci. Med.* 9:351-63.

Navarro, V. 1976. *Medicine under Capitalism*. New York: Prodist.

Richmond, J. 1981. Health Behavior and Public Policy. Address, Harvard Medical School.

Stevens, R. 1971. *American Medicine and the Public Interest*. New Haven, Conn.: Yale University Press.

Szasz, T. 1961. *The Myth of Mental Illness*. New York: Delta.

Unschuld, P. U. 1975. Medico-Cultural Conflicts in Asian Settings: An Explanatory Theory. *Soc. Sci. Med.* 9:303-12.

_____. 1979. *Medical Ethics in Imperial China*. Berkeley: University of California Press.

PART I

Medical Systems and the Nature of Medicalization

Medical systems are subsystems within the general system of a society. As such systems, they are potentially competitive with other subsystems for available resources. To the extent that they are discrete entities, medical systems may rise, come to power, hold corporate social identities, and fall. The dynamics of medical activity in the social system provide one definition of medicalization. In the chapters that follow, the authors offer varying points of view about the evolution, behavior, consequences, and context of medical system activities.

In Chapter 1, Janzen introduces a comparative perspective and stresses the need for a scholarly and cross-cultural analysis of the medicalization concept. He distinguishes taxonomic and political aspects of medicine's role. Tracing alterations in the Western taxonomic system, or medical vocabulary, from the Galenic to the present, he notes a continual *narrowing* of disease notions. With the advent of anatomically defined disease categories, the role of medicine as a guide or standard for living vanished. Janzen concludes that medicalization more reflects the usurpation of medical activities by state and professional bureaucracies than an expansion of taxonomic control by the medical system itself. When compared with the taxonomic system of Bantu Africa, Janzen views the attempt by medicine to break out of the "straight jacket medical paradigm" that so constrains Western practitioners as the stimulus for the medicalization debate.

Fabrega discusses the evolution of medical systems from elementary societies to the present and suggests a course of increasing differentiation, specialization, and independence from other systems in the social network (Chapter 2). Medicine's independence is an important differentiating feature and has allowed it to influence strongly larger society. Fabrega, however, stresses the limits of the heuristic notion that the medical system is cleaved from the general organization of society. Instead, he argues that health and disease concerns are pervasive across subsystems in society. He considers the perspective of certain critics that society is a normative scheme with discretely bounded social institutions and functions that are naive and incorrect. Accordingly, Fabrega argues, based on the interconnectedness of illness and social experience, against the split between the social and the medical. He views medicalization and socialization as inseparable.

On the other hand, Lasch, in Chapter 3, argues against the helpfulness of cross-cultural comparisons for elucidating the issue of medicalization. He sees it as occurring in the specific historical configuration of the West. Lasch argues against the conspiratorial notion of medicalization and stresses its entanglements with the historical ascendancy of the therapeutic and professional class. A triumph of the therapeutic class is that it has encouraged an atrophy of the moral sense in the Western person and social system. These changes have led medicine into maintaining a client state in which the medical model has been generalized into programs for social improvement and engineering.

In Chapter 4, Kleinman agrees that medicalization in the West is distinctive but argues for a more complex understanding of medicalization that takes into account the nature of medical systems as cultural systems. Medical systems have three subsectors: (1) the professional, (2) the folk, and (3) the lay. The fact that medicalization may occur in each of these subsectors is what leads to the complexity of the medicalization process. Kleinman points out that 70-90 percent of world health care is carried out in the lay subsector and that an exclusive focus on the professional sector, by a historical analysis limited to one culture, can minimize the importance of medicalization as an analytical tool. He stresses that medicalization is not wrongheaded or maladaptive and suggests restraint on the part of our social science colleagues so that the notion is not trivialized by shallow criticism. Kleinman views the medicalization idea as a fertile source for hypothesis formation that may be tested historically and cross-culturally.

1

MEDICALIZATION IN COMPARATIVE PERSPECTIVE

John M. Janzen

A scholarly consideration of "medicalization" or "overmedicalization" calls for some method of objective assessment of the degree of medicalization that has occurred in Western medicine. Critiques by Illich, Szasz, and others allege a process of expansion of "the medical" or control by medical professionals. They present a very shallow perspective, usually limited to the United States and to the past few decades (Illich, 1976; Szasz, 1961; Waitzkin and Waterman, 1974). The historical scope of an investigation of medicalization needs to be extended back at least to the sixteenth century for a comparison with the premodern paradigm of Greek (or Galenic) humoral medicine that then reigned supreme. Although historians of medicine can do this well, the comparative integral dimension is needed, necessitating an anthropological contribution. In addition, comparisons should be made with non-Western traditions to offer understanding of different medical paradigms that "medicalize" life's domains in other ways and to greater or lesser degree than does our own. The particular comparative case I know best is that of the societies of Bantu Africa. The comparison is pertinent because this medical tradition is an important source for cultural (and medical) pluralism in the Americas. Bantu African medicine is unique and systematic. A study of Western medicine's encounter with it permits clear contrasts to emerge.

A comparison of modern medicine in the West with its own past and with the Bantu African medical system should first establish the nature of causality in each system, look at the classification of phenomena fitted into categories of affliction and therapy, and establish the nature of the medical system's social structure, the control of resources used in therapy, and the norms, organizations, and codes shaping the careers of practitioners.

The comparative agenda thus identifies cultural matters, which give content to the medical system, and social matters, which give it shape and strength and indicate the degree of control it exercises on the society. This should make possible a more objective discussion of medicalization in modern medicine.

GALENIC WESTERN MEDICINE AND THE MODERN SCIENTIFIC PARADIGM

The understanding of disease and health in Greek antiquity developed around the imbalance and balance of humors and natural elements. It reached a high point in the work of Paracelsus (1493-1540), an early Renaissance medical practitioner and scholar. His medical cosmology pivoted on the importance of natural powers of creation and dissolution and on the related regions of human morality; it was a total life system.

From Paracelsus, Western medicine has narrowed down its causal and classificatory domains of disease and health. Vesalius (1514-1564), for example, in his study of anatomy, shifted the focus of medicine away from the cosmos to the human body. As a result of his work, physiology, pathology, and physical diagnosis became standard and specialized traditions of inquiry in which subsequent figures would develop, and further narrow, the scope of medical taxonomies (Hudson, 1978). Later medical scholars (e.g., Margagni in the early eighteenth century) rejected "fluids" in the body as the seat of disease, emphasizing instead organs and organisms as the unit of the human anatomy susceptible to disease and therefore needing treatment. Virchow (1821-1902) further localized anatomy to the study of tissue. Medical historians have generally agreed that this progressive narrowing of the focus of anatomy and physiology continues, historically, right into the present when medical scholarship entails analysis of cells, molecules, and atoms — ever smaller, more "elemental" units.

The Western history of disease conceptualization follows a similar path, from that of the human person constituting a miniature reflection of the whole cosmos to the understanding of disease as an alien object within the human body.

Sydenham (1624-1689), physician and close friend of empiricist philosopher John Locke, studied (malarial) "recurrent fever." Sydenham posited the existence of a specific disease entity. He is often identified as a critical figure in the transition to Western medicine and the understanding of disease as an observable thing and causally as a single identifiable intruding agent. Here, as in anatomy and physiology, medical historians tend to see a lineal unfolding of an explanatory model in later centuries, particularly that represented by the infectious diseases that gave rise to the modern bacteriology of Pasteur, Koch, and Jenner and the isolation of the great contagious diseases (Hudson, 1978).

The line of historical reconstruction I have followed thus far in tracing the transformation of Western medicine from the broad Galenic paradigm of humors to the narrow paradigm of bodily organs and intrusive disease agents is essentially an intellectual history, concentrating on theories of causality and the scope of taxonomies. Medical historians atuned to social forces are not satisfied that such broad transformations as occurred in Western medicine from the sixteenth to the eighteenth centuries can be fully explained by intellectual paradigms.

One area of recent scholarship — medical history as social history — has sought to account for the impact of Sydenham's disease model in English medicine in terms of social forces of the seventeenth century, the century of the English revolution (Feierman, 1979). It is argued that ideas are not sufficient in themselves to transform institutions and thus establish scientific traditions; such ideas must be defended and promoted by social groups and classes and by ruling elites and governments. Not only were the popular classes prompted by revolutionary thought to abandon the various alternative "medicines" of astrology, witchcraft, and spiritism, but, more importantly, the propertied classes that defeated the revolution imposed their own regime in government and supported narrow disease-specific notions of medicine. In other words, the continuity of intellectual science was combined with a social revolution and then with a counterrevolution. A specific professional structure was imposed from above and brought about and sustained the dominance of the narrow paradigm of anatomical and intrusive disease we know as modern medicine.

It would be foolish to argue that modern medicine has persisted only because it was promoted by the ruling classes. The dramatic victories attributed to this narrow disease model over scourge after scourge in the late nineteenth and early twentieth centuries surely contributed to its popularity. However, it is probably correct to suggest that without support of the ruling classes and governments it could not have enjoyed access to resources it has had.

Accompanying this support, and the blessing of science, has come the development of the total medical institution, the centralized hospital (Foucault, 1961, 1963). With this has come the helplessness of the patient. Without wishing to insist overly on any element of the "modern medical system," it does appear to be a system of cohering, interdependent characteristics. These include narrow, localized anatomical causality, intrusive objectified disease theory, and the isolation of the individual (McQueen, 1978). The social dimensions that frequently accompany the above cultural features are the centralized, asylumlike institution of treatment and support by a professional or a governmental elite. All of these together, and the recent embrace of technological medicine (Reiser, 1978; Moser, 1969), have no doubt contributed to the high iatrogenic (i.e., medically caused) disease effect. But the questions remain: which characteristics of this modern medical system, as described here, are central to it, and which are peripheral or accidental? Does it tend to be institutionally centralized because it happens often to be supported by ruling elites who enjoy its benefits? Or must it be centralized because of its unique, narrow anatomical paradigm?

There is one remaining medical historical explanation accompanying the Sydenham transition to narrow disease theory. This comes from a medical historian who has been confronted with comparative medical systems and who has sought to come to grips with questions such as the foregoing. According to Bates (1978), the Sydenham shift in medical explanation constituted less a change of paradigm than an "impoverishment of taxonomy" in orthodox medicine. Medical practice continued on an empirical basis, but medical theory did not replace, in kind, the systemic quality of Galenic medicine, especially not in the close relationship between the natural and the moral world found in Paracelsus' work. Bates suggests that this impoverishment of modern medicine's taxonomy accounts for the inability of Western modern medicine to displace local medical systems the world over. I would argue that this inability to displace due to impoverishment is the reason Western medicine must usually be structured in an authoritarian, centralized social framework to survive. One could test Bates' supposition by examining those societies in the world in which Galenic medicine, or some variant within it, such as Yunani, has survived to the present and into which society modern medicine has been introduced. Data from Central America, and especially from Mexico, would be interesting in this regard (Vargas, 1978). In Asia there are numerous settings, such as Iran and India, where Greek-Arab medicine survives alongside modern medicine (Leslie, 1976).

Another case that has come to my attention is that of Tunisia, where fieldwork by Teitelbaum has identified clearly the cultural and the social facts of the interpenetration of Greek and modern medicine on a case-specific basis. In an article on the social perception of illness in Tunisia, Teitelbaum (1975) describes how modern medicine is well represented by French and Tunisian medical doctors, who are widely consulted for their reputed skills in healing; however, most of the society utilizes humoral theory to understand its own illnesses. Furthermore, few if any humoral practitioners of professional stature are found in the society. A central idea in the causality of affliction in Tunisian humoral medicine is that worry and anger (i.e., social conflict) will lead to plethora, the lack of or "rotting" blood or "black" blood. This will further lead to weakness and "heartbreak." These all express the imbalance of the humors. Traditional therapy prescribes mystical acts, magical foods, and bleeding in order to cleanse the blood. Visitation and reconciliation may achieve good health without physical intervention. Modern medical care may substitute at times for humoral therapies; it is widely sought in terms of specific infections and ailments. French private practitioners are preferred over the free government-sponsored clinics. Still, these specific cures sought in modern medical facilities are always contextualized within the general rubrics of humoral and moral concepts. Teitelbaum observes, "In health matters villagers look toward the most advanced medical aids and have recourse to traditional cures simultaneously" (1975, p. 402). Such a mix works, in terms of the logic of therapeutic systems, because humoral medicine has no germ theory and modern medicine has no moral theory. Humoral medicine situates the individual within a broader social and cosmic whole and prescribes a condition of moral order that restores balanced humors in the body. Modern medicine offers demonstrable relief for specific physical ailments but no guide or standard for living in human society.

The Tunisian example, as well as the seventeenth century transition of medicine around the ideas of Sydenham, suggests that the modern medical paradigm may persist only where it has the backing of a professional elite and government, because its taxonomy of health is impoverished. Classical Galenic humoral medicine survives without practitioners because its taxonomy offers an active concept of health, namely balance and harmony.

The comparisons suggest something about medicalization as well. The medicalization critique of modern medicine makes no sense as strictly applied to its taxonomic and causal dimensions, since these are the most specific and narrow the world has ever seen. The critique of political domination, as medicalization, makes far more sense, since social domination has often, apparently, been a feature of modern medicine. The implications of this realization — that the most medicalized system thrives even without practitioners and the narrow medical taxonomy requires practitioner domination and total institutional frameworks — need to be deferred until another comparison is made: between modern medicine and Bantu African medicine.

MODERN MEDICINE IN BANTU AFRICA

The conclusions reached by turning modern medicine — culturally and socially — back on its own past may be tested further by comparing it with a rather different medicine such as that of Bantu Africa, a medical-cultural tradition perhaps a thousand years old that possesses a high degree of conceptual and institutional development although not the textual tradition of intellectual history. Nevertheless, intellectual sophistication is present since recognizable ideas have survived in emigrant African cultures in Brazil, Mexico, the Caribbean, and the United States (Bastide, 1967).

The causal system of health and disease in Bantu thought traces all of life to a central source of power such as God or nature. This power is mediated by middle-range spirits and consecrated human priests, who maintain the ideal of retaining contact with, or inspiration from, the source of power and life. Evil, including disease, is any condition, be it social, personal, physical, or mystical that falls short of the ordered universe of life. Balance between the universe's elements is a subordinate theme, as is purity.

A crucial cosmological notion is the distinction drawn in all Bantu societies between naturally caused (or God-caused) disease and misfortune and that attributed to human cause (Orley, 1970; Turner, 1968; Swantz, 1970; Ngubane, 1977; Feierman, 1979; Janzen, 1978b). Naturally caused disease "just happens" (Ngubane, 1977) or is "in the order of things," for example, the death of a very old person or an affliction with readily recognized symptoms and signs that heals as expected. A widespread range of treatments, such as plant preparations, massages, and manipulative techniques, are appropriate for afflictions of this type, as are the techniques of modern medicine practiced by Western-trained doctors and nurses in hospitals and dispensaries.

In contrast to natural diseases are those caused by chaos in the human world or in the relationship of humans to their environment. An individual may develop suffering and disease by disregarding social etiquette, by ignoring good eating habits, or by ignoring kinsmen, elders, ancestors, and spirits. An aura of ritual pollution frequently accompanies sickness by "human cause," requiring the sufferer to seek ritual purification through sacrifices and confessions so as to achieve reintegration to the good graces of society (Ngubane, 1977; Douglas, 1966). Most human-caused affliction in Bantu thought is attributed to evil intentions of others or to situations of contradiction in which people are at odds or cross purposes with one another, for example, in a struggle to distribute land equitably from a bounded estate at a time when the dependent population is increasing or in launching an enterprise for profit in the face of a strong ethic advocating the redistribution of goods. Such situations are believed to incur the ill will or envy of others and to lead directly to the breakdown of health in a person, to visible physical sickness, or to death. This belief in mystically channeled ill wishing operates to reinforce the morality of social redistribution and loyalty to family and kin.

Flowing from these assumptions about the nature of the world and the causes of misfortune, Bantu medical systems articulate therapeutic techniques — empirical, social, symbolical — and their appropriate specialists. Not all such "medicines" are specialized knowledge, of course. Many are common household techniques, practiced by mothers and fathers on their children or in self-treatment. In areas of life relating to crisis, transition, danger, recurrent accident, high responsibility, or core social values, there arise consecrated medicines, with origin charters, exact codes for their use, and dangers of their misuse. These consecrated medicines may be techniques, chemotherapeutic treatments, behavioral procedures, or highly magical and esoteric affairs. Examples will be given below. The above-mentioned dichotomy of natural afflictions and human-caused afflictions is not to be confused with the distinction between common "secular" therapeutic techniques and somewhat specialized consecrated medicines. The emergence of a consecrated medicine in an area of life, with its charter, ownership, and unique ritual, probably derives from the perception that it is powerful, effective, and therefore in need of legitimate control. In the words of one Kongo writer, "a medicine that can kill, can also cure"; therefore, it must be carefully used and authorized (Kusikila, 1966). This is no different from the legitimation process for medicines and specialists in other medical systems. Western medicine in Bantu society is given the status of consecrated medicine; its healers are called *banganga* and are imbued with magical powers.

Generally, then, a Bantu medical system is organized into a series of *nganga* specialist types (plural, *banganga*), each of whom has received instruction in, or initiation to, one or more consecrated medicines. Among the BaKongo, classically, the *nganga mbuki* (from *buka*, "to heal") would be a local doctor. The *nganga n'kisi* is a more advanced or specialized doctor competent in numerous consecrated medicines, especially those pertaining to anger and magically caused afflictions. The *nganga ngombo* (named after the basket he uses) is the diviner, a type widespread across Bantu Africa, whose specialty is the sorting out of particular features in cases and the offering of an expert diagnosis of the affliction or misfortune's cause, whether it be of natural or human cause or of other spirit-related cause. Because of its integral place in the analysis and interpretation of human experience in Bantu society, divination has responded sensitively, as an institution, to social change. Particular perspectives in divination have come and gone; inspirational diviners and prophet-seers, even mission-trained pastors and priests, have taken on the role in the past century. Where traditional, precolonial diviners have disappeared as a specialized type of *nganga*, kinsmen of sufferers and prophet-seers do this work. Yet Bantu divination, as a social process, has remained strong, explaining the remarkable resilience of Bantu medicine and its ability to generate new consecrated medicines — surface transformations — without changing basic premises.

In most local Bantu medical systems, a few of the consecrated medicines take on public status as "drums" or "cults" of affliction (see Chapter 10). These are characterized by a membership consisting of fellow sufferers of a common affliction, organized into local chapters. Bantu drums of affliction share the feature that those afflicted, and cured or stabilized in their relationship to the sickness, are the best suited to become specialized doctors of the particular ailment for which the drum is known. Sickness is seen as a sacred calling; often its manifestation is a form of possession. If the possessing sickness or its emanating spirit is placated and the disease is conquered, the sickness purifies and energizes the individual. Thus the individual owes a debt to society and is expected to consecrate the newly found gifts as a medium of ultimate power in this specialized domain and to serve others. (These are discussed further in Chapter 2.)

The foregoing is a standardized picture of Bantu medicine, for which there are local variants and historical viscissitudes. In times of rapid change or crisis, well-defined "drum" associations dissolve, replaced by ephemeral movements symptomatic of the troubling issues facing the society (DeCraemer, Vansina, and Fox, 1977). Where stable, centralized polities are found, drums tend to be fewer in number, or absent altogether, their function having been subsumed under centralized state orders. Elsewhere I have discussed the distinction between major permanent drums of affliction representing a society's normative structure and ephemeral drums or medicines in terms of differential group incorporatedness (Janzen, 1978a). The former have full corporate group status; the latter are often only corporate categories or movements. In any event, the various medicines, consecrated medicines, and drums of affliction (i.e., superconsecrated medicines) wax and wane, offering the scholar a clear indicator of sociocultural stability and of the contours of medicalization.

A Kongo writer of the turn of the century developed an inventory of consecrated medicines (therapeutic techniques) in his society, including the following areas of concern: "personal physical growth," "a child's upbringing," "spirit children and how to deal with them," "twinship and parenting of twins," "headache," "purification with cupping horn," "divination" (eight kinds), "clan leadership," "chiefship," "origin, residence, identity," "relating to water spirits," "order of markets and public sites," "judicial affairs," and so on. Of these, those relating to judicial affairs, clan leadership, chiefship, and order in public places were drums of affliction, that is, corporate orders. A number more pertained to women's troubles, but the author, a man, wrote nothing on these (Nsemi, 1974).

Another Kongo inventory of more recent origin lists the major consecrated medicines (*min'kisi*) to which an *nganga ngombo* diviner may refer sufferers and their clients, including the treatment of the following: "headache," "mouth diseases," "skin diseases and eruptions," "excessive menstrual bleeding," "illnesses among young women," "instilling or terminating pregnancy," "removing impurities by use of cupping horn," "insanity," "women's sterility," "childbirth troubles," "consecration of clan chiefship," and "calming villages and the countryside" (Fu-kiau, 1969). Note that these lists include specific physical afflictions and their treatments, as well as those that are highly political and public. The medicalization of life is extreme by any criterion Illich has mentioned; yet there is a difference between this medicalization and that Illich describes.

Turner offers perhaps the most extensive inventory of drums of affliction from any Bantu people, the Ndembu of Zambia, a southern Lunda group (Turner, 1968). Numerous drums pertain to hunting, the major activity of men, with such afflictions as "ancestral shades chasing the game away," "animals not appearing," "hunters persistently failing to find game," "hunters missing aim through trembling," "hunters failing to kill animals," and the like. Other drums exist among the Ndembu for "respiratory disorders," "severe and sudden illnesses," "witchcraft or sorcery-caused illness," "wasting away," "sores and boils on feet," "reproductive troubles," "leprosy," and "crop failure." Reproductive cults are specialized in terms of "menstrual disorders," "barrenness," "miscarriages," "ill health of infants," "abortions," "twin pregnancies," "delayed birth," and the like. In addition to its surprising high number of drum associations, Turner's accounts reveal that the colonial experience is dealt with by the Ndembu by channeling troubles held to be caused by dreams of Europeans, speaking with tongues simulating Europeans, and symptoms such as respiratory disorders or wasting away, probably a reflection of tuberculosis, and barrenness, reflecting venereal diseases (Prins, 1979).

A final inventory of medicines (called "charms" by these authors) is taken from the heart of colonialism, a Belgian government file in Kananga, Zaire, reflecting movements considered subversive by the colonial government (DeCraemer, Vansina, and Fox, 1977). It reflects the same broad taxonomy of problem areas as in the foregoing inventories but more of the ephemeral movement character. Present in the list are the standard themes of "women's fertility," "general health," and "global well-being." Other themes suggest the strong deisre to live effectively, in such terms as "successful hunt," "abundant harvest," "material wealth and prosperity," "to get ahead in status and prestige," and "success in undertakings." A number are distinctly anticolonial, focusing on themes such as "impunity vis-à-vis the authorities," "to become like a European," "to replace Europeans," "liberty, independence," "vengeance with impunity," and "success in war." Others address spiritual well-being in terms such as "Africanization of Christianity," "return of a golden age," "salvation," and "protection against evil, sorcery and witchcraft."

When modern Western medicine was introduced into Bantu societies in the twentieth century, diviners and lay "therapy managers" were quick to discern the areas of its competence and the nature of its classificatory focus. It became evident that modern medicine had powerful physical cures for specific diseases such as leprosy, sleeping sickness, bilharzia, smallpox, venereal diseases (except problems of infertility), and various parasites. Therefore, in some instances modern medicine replaced the work of healers whose treatments were largely specific and who used mainly herbal medicines. The clear and impressive competence of Western medicine was noted in Bantu Africa. However, in the Bantu perspective, regions of modern medicine's classificatory system had limitations. Western practitioners, for one thing, ardently denied the reality of human-caused affliction and the reality of witchcraft and sorcery. The conclusion was drawn that this general category of afflictions was not within the competency of modern medicine. The old Bantu classificatory dichotomy between natural and unnatural human-caused affliction continued to provide a standard for therapy managers in the handling of particular cases. A thorough understanding of modern medicine on the part of the lay population, nurses, and doctors in Bantu society has not appreciably altered the use of the Bantu explanatory system. In a few cases of particular diseases, such as malarial fever, now understood as being caused by mosquito carriers, or various types of infection caused by bacteria or germs, old diseases have been shifted over into the category of naturally caused, unless there are complications. However, new sources of human causation of disease have arisen. Urban life, the tensions of wage labor, job competition, political responsibility and uncertainty, and alienation, for example, have led to a need for a whole new set of specific therapies and treatments in the taxonomic zone of afflictions caused by humans. Therapy managing groups thus "shuttle" from therapies appropriate to natural illnesses to those appropriate for human-caused affliction in an effort to find the correct combination of treatments for a complex case. Often these cases involve educated elites (Janzen, 1978b). New drums of affliction are thriving in the urban centers of Bantu Africa (Corin, 1979).

DEMYTHOLOGIZING MEDICALIZATION

It has become fashionable to criticize medicalization in the Western world, even though the taxonomic expansiveness of other medical systems is ignored. Illich would have everyone be healthy; his means of achieving this is to eliminate all the iatrogenic diseases brought on by the medical establishment. If a person must suffer, then it is the individual's right to suffer alone, autonomously. As Illich puts it, "Man's consciously lived fragility, individuality, and relatedness make the experience of pain, of sickness, and of death an integral part of his life. The ability to cope with this trio autonomously is fundamental to his health" (1976, p. 272). Szasz (1961) similarly, would have the psychiatric experts redefine mental illness as a metaphorical game by those who have some reason to act sick, rather than to accept with approval the premise that hysteria, malingering, and paranoia are real mental illnesses. I understand what they are saying. But my ethnological judgment flashes a red warning light.

Evidence brought to bear on a comparative understanding of medicalization suggests that most cultural systems of medicine, including those of classical antiquity and Bantu Africa, are far more inclusive in their taxonomies of recognized affliction than that of the modern West, the end product of three centuries of narrowing down of the medical taxonomy to a mechanized, atomized, and materialized concept of the human being. And yet Illich and Szasz launch their attack from within this individualistic framework. Instead of evaluating, they are calling for the positivistic reification of the received categories! If we take them literally, they would eliminate what meager legitimation still exists in illness categories. The belief that somehow health would result from the elimination of the labeling and treating system I cannot comprehend. Does our modern industrial life have no ailments, then? Is the only option that of valiantly suffering, alone? No, the critique of medicalization makes no sense as a critique of taxonomic overextension.

The real, and only, validity of the medicalization critique is these political questions: who controls medical culture, seen in terms of the legitimate right to label illness and disease; who has the (exclusive) right to treat; and what should the prestige be of practitioners in exercising these rights (Unschuld, 1975)? In this respect the evidence is overwhelming that professional or state bureaucracies control the healing resources. In the United States the former do; in some other countries the latter do.

Critics of medicalization would "deregulate" the medical resource. But there is a problem in this line of analysis. These critics wish to eliminate the medical bureaucracy and the medical elite, but they remain intent on keeping a very narrow illness taxonomy, a literal one that does not invent or fictionalize iatrogenic diseases. The seventeenth century emergence of "narrow" medicine, and the subsequent introduction of this medicine into other systems, suggests that a medical system as narrow in focus as this — physicalized, atomized, materialized, individualized, mechanized, and curative — can be maintained only by an external elite that controls the "reality" of what constitutes a disease and codes that license practitioners.

Surely, once the professional, state-supported, medical elite would be decontrolled or eliminated, categories of disease and therapy would proliferate to social and religious domains. Put another way, a proliferated, socially embedded disease taxonomy of the type seen by Paracelsus, in modern folk Tunisian humoral medicine, or in Bantu African medicine precludes centralized control.

It is unlikely that the professional stronghold of dominant medicine in the United States will be broken in the near future. The ruling medicine continues to be effective in many physical diseases despite the iatrogenic diseases it invents or produces. Furthermore, it is clear that Western industrial society has the equivalent of Bantu diseases of human origin, as well as a myriad of nonprofessional social therapies to deal with them (see Chapter 10).

Critics of medicalization offer no effective analysis for the real ills of modern society. Rather than to mystify the narrow paradigm of a scientific elite of medics by recommending an even narrower paradigm, they should offer us genuine critiques of industrial society and the means of living in it. Why, indeed, do people invent hysterias, malingering, paranoias, and neuroses? Autonomy will not cure whatever ills our society imposes on us. I suspect we have too much individual autonomy already.

Mitscherlich's (1966, 1969) analysis of modern society offers such a picture of our afflictions. His writing on social conflict states that psychosomatic illness demonstrates the unique conditions of human existence at a given time and place. Writing from a European philosophical anthropology of medicine, he sees such illness as a profile of how a person loses or denies individual freedom. In this his thinking is comparable to that of Illich and Szasz; an effort to discover the self is often rewarded by actual healing and the return of health. With them, he states that this process of finding the self inalienably is accompanied by human suffering. He departs from them in his assertion that therapeutic intervention may achieve, and ideally should achieve, the transformation of senseless sickness, which is the denial of freedom, into meaningful suffering. Freedom is thus won through an acknowledgement of conflict and human suffering − an assertion of the sacredness of suffering. With this, Mitscherlich begins to sound like a theoretician of a Bantu drum or a Euroamerican anonymous society such as Alcoholics Anonymous. Indeed, Mitscherlich's inventory of pressing problems in modern society in need of attention resembles the inventories listed above from Bantu Africa: "stresses of achievement"; "the bureaucratization (compartmentalization) of life"; "the destruction of the urban environment and of ecological equilibrium"; "problems of motivation and education"; and "the invasion of forms of economic and administrative rationality into areas of life in which the latitude for choice − play, freedom − has been diminished, areas such as self expression, training for morality and practical action, aesthetic satisfaction and spontaneity"; also, "impulses for critical judgement, the renewal of tradition, and the creation of new perspectives become ever weaker" (Habermas, 1978). These are the conflicts, the sources of illness, that are typical of our time and that any critique of medicalization must take into account and from which it must begin its analysis.

REFERENCES

Bastide, R. 1967. *Les Amériques Noires: Les Civilisations Africaines dans le Nouveau Monde*. Paris: Payot.

Bates, D. 1978. Comments to panel on History of African Pluralistic Medical Systems. Baltimore: African Studies Association.

Corin, E. 1979. A Possession Psychotherapy in an Urban Setting: Zebola in Kinshasa. In *The Social History of Disease and Medicine in Africa*, ed. J. M. Janzen and S. Feierman, pp. 327-38. Oxford: Pergamon. Special Issue *Soc. Sci. Med.* 13B(no. 4).

DeCraemer, W., Vansina, J., and Fox, R. 1977. Religious Movements in Central Africa: A Theoretical Study. *Comp. Studies Society History* 18:458-75.

Douglas, M. 1966. *Purity and Danger: An Analysis of Concepts of Pollution and Taboo*. New York: Praeger.

Feierman, S. 1979. Change in African Therapeutic Systems. In *The Social History of Disease and Medicine in Africa*, ed. J. M. Janzen and S. Feierman, pp. 277-84. Oxford: Pergamon. Special Issue *Soc. Sci. Med.* 13B (no. 4).

Foucault, M. 1961. *Histoire de la Folie*. Paris: Plon.

———. 1963. *Naissance de la Clinique*. Paris: Presses Universitaries de France.

Fu-Kiau kia Bunseki-Lumanisa. 1969. *Kindoki, ou la Solution Attendue*. Kumba: Académie Kongolaise.

Habermas, J. 1978. Arzt und Intellektuller: Alexander Mitscherlich zum 70. Geburtstag. *Die Zeit* 39.

Hudson, R. 1978. Lecture in History of Medicine. Lawrence: University of Kansas.

Illich, I. 1976. *Medical Nemesis: The Expropriation of Health*. New York: Pantheon.

Janzen, J. M. 1978a. The Comparative Study of Medical Systems as Changing Social Systems. In *Theoretical Foundations for the Comparative Study of Medical Systems*, ed. C. Leslie, pp. 121-29. Oxford: Pergamon. Special Issue *Soc. Sci. Med.* 12 (no. 2B).

———. 1978b. *The Quest for Therapy in Lower Zaire*. Berkeley: University of California Press.

———. 1979. Ideologies and Institutions in the Precolonial History of Equatorial African Therapeutic Systems. In *The Social History of Disease and Medicine in Africa*, ed. J. M. Janzen and S. Feierman, pp. 317-26. Oxford: Pergamon. Special Issue *Soc. Sci. Med.* 13B(no. 4).

Janzen, J. M., and MacGaffey, W. 1974. *Anthology of Kongo Religion*. Lawrence: University of Kansas Publications in Anthropology 5.

Janzen, J. M., and Feierman, S. 1979. *The Social History of Disease and Medicine in Africa*. Oxford: Pergamon. Special Issue *Soc. Sci. Med.* 13B(no. 4).

Kusikila-kwa-Kilombo. 1966. *Lufwa evo Kimongi e?* Kumba: Académie Kongolaise.

Leslie, C. 1976. *Asian Medical Systems*. Berkeley: University of California Press.

McQueen, D. 1978. The History of Science and Medicine as Theoretical Sources for the Comparative Study of Contemporary Medical Systems. In *Theoretical Foundations for the Comparative Study of Medical Systems*, ed. C. Leslie, pp. 69-74. Oxford: Pergamon. Special Issue *Soc. Sci. Med.* 12(no. 2B).

Mitscherlich, A. 1966, 1969. *Krankheit als Konflikt: Studien zur Psychosomatischen Medizin*. Frankfurt am Main: Suhrkamp.

Moser, 1969. *The Disease of Medical Progress: A Study of Iatrogenic Disease*. Springfield, Ill.: Thomas.

Ngubane, H. 1977. *Body and Mind in Zulu Medicine*. New York: Academic Press.

Nsemi, I., 1974. Min'kisi: Sacred Medicines. In *Anthology of Kongo Religion*, ed. J. M. Janzen and W. MacGaffey, pp. 34-38. Lawrence: University of Kansas Publications in Anthropology 5.

Orley, J. 1970. African Medical Taxonomy. *J. Anthropol. Society Oxford* 1(3):137-50.

Prins, G. 1979. Disease at the Crossroads: Towards a History of Therapeutics in Bulozi since 1876. In *The Social History of Disease and Medicine in Africa*, ed. J. M. Janzen and S. Feierman, pp. 285-316. Oxford: Pergamon. Special Issue *Soc. Sci. Med.* 13B(no. 4).

Reiser, S. J. 1978. *Medicine and the Reign of Technology*. Cambridge: Cambridge University Press.

Swantz, M. 1970. *Ritual and Symbol in Transitional Zaramo Society*. Uppsala: Gleerup.

Szasz, T. 1961. *The Myth of Mental Illness*. New York: Delta.

Teitelbaum, J. M. 1975. The Social Perception of Illness in Some Tunisian Villages. In *Psychological Anthropology*, ed. T. R. Williams, pp. 401-8. The Hague: Mouton.

Turner, V. W. 1968. *Drums of Affliction*. Oxford: Clarendon.

Unschuld, P. 1975. Medico-cultural Conflicts in Asian Settings. *Soc. Sci. Med.* 9:303-12.

Vargas, L. 1978. Lecture on Medical History and Anthropology in Mexico. Lawrence: University of Kansas.

Waitzkin, H. B., and Waterman, B. 1974. *The Exploitation of Illness in Capitalist Society*. New York: Bobbs-Merrill.

2

THE IDEA OF MEDICALIZATION:
An Anthropological Perspective

Horacio Fabrega, Jr.

The idea that medicalization is taking place in contemporary society seems to imply that attitudes and concerns that properly
should be directed at "medical" problems are being misdirected to
phenomena or problems of a different character altogether. Individuals who speak of medicalization seem to have in mind a more or
less normative picture of society and judge that particular types of
problems can be clearly bounded, labeled unproblematically, and
dealt with through delimitable institutions of control. Such individuals often follow a historical and comparative point of view
and have in mind a previous era when the domain of disease-illness
and medical care was more "correctly" interpreted.

The idea of medicalization is not widely used by anthropologists
who study medical phenomena in preliterate and literate societies.
All anthropologists, especially biologically oriented ones, would
agree that the concrete physical changes in the body that are seen
today and linked to disease are ubiquitous and recurring and have
been the lot of humanity throughout the period of human evolution. Moreover, all anthropologists, especially culturally oriented
ones, would support the idea that peoples of the world differ greatly
in the way they define disease-illness and go about dealing with
the problems linked to this. The latter type of anthropologist would
probably challenge the assumption that there is a distinct and
more or less correct view of disease-illness and medical care, an

assumption central to historians, sociologists, and social critics who endorse the idea of medicalization (Illich, 1976; Lasch, 1977).

In this chapter the idea of medicalization is analyzed from a general anthropological point of view. The way in which medical problems are handled in preliterate societies is given principal attention, although material from the social history of Western medicine is included. Relations between medicine and society are looked at culturally and also from an evolutionary point of view. This type of approach should allow one to look at the problem of "medicalization" in a broader way.

ILLNESS AND DISEASE IN A GENERAL ANTHROPOLOGICAL FRAME OF REFERENCE

Things we describe as "illness" and "disease" are universal happenings in social groups. All peoples, it seems, experience disease and illness and want to be rid of them. Disease and illness are also universal biological phenomenon. The conditions for disease-illness are prescribed by the synthetic theory of evolution. This is to say that key concepts of evolutionary biology, such as genetic variability, environment, adaptation, and natural selection, are sufficient to explain occurrences of illness and disease. In a strict biological evolutionary sense, disease-illness is a factor that influences the operation of natural selection. It is one of the sources of adaptive variability that determines which organisms are selected; and if genetic factors underlie the disease-illness (in evolutionary theory, the expression of a poor organism-environment fit), these will be underrepresented in future generations (Fabrega, 1975).

Anthropologists emphasize the social dimension of an individual's medical problem (Fabrega, 1979). They often use the term "illness" in a special way to emphasize a disvalued state or condition of the individual considered as a whole being. By illness they meant something manifested concretely in behavior adaptation, and they draw a distinction between this and the underlying disorder or disease process, which is physical. Illness is thus construed as a discontinuity in the life arc of a person, involving an impairment in function and hence a deviation. In all groups, a state of illness is associated with a relative failure to perform basic expected tasks. The individual acknowledges — implicitly or explicitly — an "ill" state and shows this overtly in behavior, covertly, or symbolically in words. The social group usually validates or certifies a claim of illness. This is a fairly general observation, although it is not true in our culture. Our system of medicine allows positing that someone who claims illness is really not physically diseased. A malingerer, for example, is a person claiming illness who is judged as not diseased by a physician. In an anthropological sense, the acknowledgment or judgment by individuals that they are ill is usually sufficient to qualify them for the social state of illness. However, this need not be true, for in all cultures, people with so-called mental illness often are judged by co-members as ill, although they themselves may not necessarily see themselves as ill.

The cultural orientation of the person and of the group plays a critical role in how illness will be interpreted, explained, responded to, and dealt with — that is, the meaning given to illness. An episode of illness does not contain this, for an illness is essentially a state of impairment in well-being. The people's culture or system of social symbols and their meanings furnish the name, explanation, and treatment rationale for an illness. The raw material is a person showing dysfunction, often linked to bodily changes. There may be universal and generic physical changes underlying this. Even these, however, we read into the illness picture by means of our scientific conventions. This means that the personal belief as to how an individual is constructed or formed (the view of self) will influence how the individual reports or explains the illness and treats it. Thus, in an anthropological sense, a people's theory of personhood and its theory of illness are locked together and influence illness behavior and explanation in a fundamental way. All societies have such culturally specific theories about why people behave the way they do, why and how they get ill, how illness changes the person, and what being ill implies about the person. Two key propositions of our (Western) theory of personhood and theory of illness are the "bodily" (i.e., physical) as opposed to the "mental" (the locus of volition), and "illnesses are traceable to physical *disease* processes or disorders of the body."

SOCIAL-ECOLOGICAL CONDITIONS OF PHYSICAL STATES OF DISEASE

An assumption of the physical anthropologist is that the biological characteristics of humans were forged in a simplified, elementary form of social organization. This type of social group was probably standard during human evolution. Groups classified as elementary, or bands, are small and migratory and their members are highly inter-dependent; environmental pressures are jointly experienced. All facets of human life have a social and shared basis. The effects of disease viewed as a physical condition, then, are visible to co-members, and the latter share in the tribulations of those who are ill. In such social settings, an occurrence of disease does not simply incapacitate or eliminate an individual in some mechanical sense. Rather, it affects the individual's capacity and performance as a participating member of a highly interdependent group. Only at this point, when it comes to affect the behavior of an individual, does disease assume relevance as a biological phenomenon. As indicated earlier, this important behavioral dimension of disease is a reason for the widespread use of the idea of illness.

With regard to biological sources of illness among elementary societies, the following ten generalizations can be offered (Boyden, 1970):

1. Illnesses among these people were importantly influenced by exposures to infections with microorganisms and parasites common to the animals with which they came into direct contact.

2. What are termed today typically human immunities, which have no apparent animal reservoir (e.g., polio, measles, influenza), were probably nonexistent among elementary groupings because the respective microorganisms require a large enough human popula-tion to provide a pool of noninfected susceptibles and the size of bands was simply too small for this.

3. Infections characterized by a longer latency, marked by recurrence, which were essentially chronic and in which reinfection was possible, provided a large proportion of the conditions of the forms of disease found among elementary groupings.

4. Infections that could be propagated vertically across gener-ations (which meant a symbiotic relation between agent and infected host) may have been prominent.

5. The diet of the poor is composed of highly palatable items that yield highly refined carbohydrate sources, and this has suggested to many that the conditions for caries and obesity may have been less prevalent.

6. Life was physically demanding, the level of activity was high, obesity was probably uncommon, but leisure time for group activity was ample; these conditions may have involved fewer changes that

are thought of today as stressful and that are believed to lead to chronic degenerative changes. Forms of illness among elementary groupings were no doubt affected by these conditions.

7. Chronic biological changes that are commonly seen in the elderly were probably rare in part because of factors already mentioned and in part because the life span of people of elementary groups was believed to be rather short for such changes to develop.

8. Deaths due to cannibalism, infanticide, sacrifice, geronticide, head hunting, and trauma were probably high among prehistorical elementary peoples.

9. Chronic skin infections were probably common.

10. Owing to the nomadic way of life, fecal-oral infection routes were not prominently implicated as factors contributing to disease forms.

With larger societies, termed "ranked," one finds more complex forms of social organization, a division of labor that extends beyond strictly sexual lines, a greater degree of role specialization, early forms of institutions, and extended interconnected families whose members are able to acquire household items and properties. With a settled form of social life, particularly when population density reaches a figure high enough to allow for microbial persistence and noninfected susceptibles (as one finds in urban settlements), comes the possibility of human epidemics (e.g., measles, smallpox). This means that these infections act as influences that can yield new illnesses for tribal groupings. Irrigation systems often mean a common water supply and hence the possibility of fecal-oral transmission, setting the stage for further changes affecting patterns of illness. Microorganisms from nondomesticated animals may be expected to have less frequently affected tribal peoples owing to their greater "distance" from a pristine physical habitat. Changing agricultural practices, however, set the stage for the rich propagation of vectors of microorganisms as well as new patterns for infection routes. Settled groupings in the absence of developed sanitary practices also means that carrier members can directly infect others through fecal-oral modes of transition. Among people of ranked societies, a diet consisting mainly of vegetable foods is a distinct possibility. Among many such groupings, however, mixed diets no doubt prevailed. Some people came to depend mainly on cereals and root crops. It is believed that a bulk of root vegetables providing around 2,500 calories complemented with significant amounts of grape leaves would have provided members of ranked societies with a nutritionally adequate diet. The bulk and water content of such diets would have yielded a slow, sustained absorption of nutrients. These features of the diet must be presumed to have affected physiologic patternings and energy balances, as well as metabolic and biochemical profiles. Since social differentiation becomes a striking feature among ranked societies, altogether different forms of personal relations may have "complicated" social life, in the process modifying the earlier familistic and egalitarian system. Social differentiation also means social inequality and more heterogeneous forms of life-styles. This, in turn, suggests that physical activity, leisure time allotments, sedentary pursuits, and a complex distribution of type and quality of food prevailed across members of a ranked social grouping. The preceding conditions must be seen as correlated with, if not producing, a higher level of individual differences in psychobiological types. This, in turn, provides sources for altogether different kinds of health profiles compared with elementary band groupings, whose members lead a much more homogeneous life.

SYSTEMS OF MEDICINE IN TWO TYPES OF SMALL-SCALE SOCIETIES

In previous publications I have described and discussed characteristics of the social orientations toward disease-illness, as well as the medical care practices of elementary and more complex (ranked) but still small-scale societies (Fabrega, in press; Fabrega and Silver, 1973). In this chapter I summarize this information and draw from it generalizations for discussion. Analyses such as these can serve as background for comparisons involving the systems of medicine of larger states and civilizations.

In both types of nonliterate groups the lay people serve as the "first line of defense" against disease-illness. Lay people share among themselves broad knowledge about medical problems and initiate treatments when symptoms arise. The responses to illness, including attempts at its treatment, are more public and visible in elementary societies, seeming to have what one could term a communal basis, whereas in more complex groups responses tend to be private and contained within the family.

In very elementary societies theories of illness draw emphasis to causal agencies and forces outside the person. Among peoples of ranked societies, although these agencies remain important, it seems to be the case that aspects of the person and "mechanisms" or "substances" within that person become more prominent in explanations of cause. This suggests that the theories of illness among ranked societies are more elaborate. In very elementary societies, medical treatment involving a practitioner tends to take place in an open setting and in a large group that includes many co-members, whereas in the more complex groups a more closed setting is preferred and the family members of the ill person are the main participants. Treatment of disease appears to be an occasion for reestablishing group "health" in elementary groups, whereas it is more individuated and focused (on the sick person and the family) in the complex groups. Family units and kin groups generally appear to be the "managers" of treatment in complex groups, whereas in elementary groups the group as a whole functions as manager.

In contrast to elementary societies, in more complex small-scale societies one finds people whose functions are clearly medical. These people possess specialized knowledge of illness and its tangible attributes. They often undergo official certification and/or have special clothing and equipment that sets them apart physically; moreover, they are highly distinguishable from co-members on social behavioral criteria. A differentiation of practitioner types exists in complex groups, each showing specialization of types of treatment (or phases of the treatment process), of illness types, or of types of causes. The possession of "worldly" knowledge about illness manifestations, mechanisms of causation, and effects of specific medicines appears to distinguish practitioners of the more complex societies. These practitioners are also known for their spiritual and preternatural expertise. However, among elementary groups, practitioners can be described as more totally concerned with purely preternatural causation and significance.

Among very elementary societies severe illnesses that require practitioner intervention appear to be judged as "undifferentiated wholes": illness behaviors subserve a general symbolic or metaphoric function, and specific manifestations and disabilities of illness are played down. Among the more complex groups, it seems, these types of illnesses appear to be judged more naturalistically, that is, their properties are judged as more differentiated, discrete, and tangible. It is possible that the actual behaviors of sick people among the more complex groups draw emphasis to types of manifestations and levels of constraints and that bodily awareness and experience are more important and diversified. Information directly supporting this is not available, although descriptions of curers' actions suggest this.

Ranked small-scale societies differ in that they tend to remunerate their medical practitioners. In most of the groups examined, the payment was considered an instrument of cure rather than a fee for the services of the curer, although the curer was personally enriched by these offerings. The curer has a broad range of power and prestige and often is relatively wealthy. What one could term a "private and materialistic" approach to medical care (i.e., contract between parties, fee for service) is observed among some of the groups studied, something that is simply not seen among the very elementary societies. In the latter, the medical practitioner seems to have little prestige, does not benefit economically from curing, and does not administer care on a private basis.

Because among ranked small-scale societies there exist specialist types of practitioners and even a hierarchy of sorts, practitioner-client relations can be said to be more focused and individuated than in elementary groups in which no differentiation exists and the group as a whole is the focus and setting of treatment. One assumes that issues of trust, obligations, bargaining, entitlements, payments or remuneration, disaffection, and dependence on the part of the patients, for example, all become significant elements of client-practitioner relations among ranked small-scale societies. In brief, among the latter, medical treatment becomes more focused, individuated, secularized, and worldly; client-practitioner relations are heightened, intensified, and made more complex; and "therapy management groups" are concerned to choose among competing interpretations about disease treatment.

POINTS OF CONTRAST WITH WESTERN CIVILIZATION

The emerging discipline of the social history of (Western) medicine provides information that one can use as a general contrast to the mode of operation of the systems of medicine of preliterate (non-Western) peoples. The striking and obvious difference is the existence of a centralized policy about health and disease and, with this, a structurally distinct social institution of medicine. This difference can be related in large part to the evolution of the state (eventually, modern civilization), which involves urbanization leading to increased size and density of populations. These social developments provided the conditions for new disease pictures linked to patterns of contagiousness. The prevalence of these new diseases, in turn, leads to social policy changes in the evolving Western system of medicine. Additional factors linked to the evolution of the Western system of medicine include (1) accumulation of written texts about disease and medicines that provide a common body of knowledge from which people and practitioner draw; (2) growth of cities, trade, and communication, educational centers, "schools of medicine," and, with this, formal education of physicians and eventually their identification as a corporate profession; (3) evolution of centralized authorities and governing bodies that increasingly come to articulate a social public health policy and to regulate licensing and eventually the practice of medicine; and (4) the emergence of science and technology, with obvious effects on understandings about disease causation, mechanisms, modes of prevention, and medical therapeutics. The above factors, together, are among the ones that constrain how illness and disease are viewed and handled in modern nations. A comparison of how modern versus nonliterate people orient to medical problems and cope with them obviously involves taking into account the instrumental-practical as well as attitudinal-cultural consequences of these demographic and sociological changes.

As an example, we may consider the effects related to the demographic transition. Especially relevant are the effects of large-scale epidemics such as those of plague and smallpox. Each of these epidemics was to some extent made possible by the new ecologies of the state civilization. Efforts linked to the control of epidemics were instrumental in fostering a "public health" orientation and, with this, the idea of state-controlled agencies with policies about health and medical care. In late Medieval-Renaissance times, centralized control and/or local governments already saw fit to create health boards empowered to institute public health measures necessitated by the then-prevailing medical problem, bubonic plague. The growth of state regulatory agencies concerned with public health problems is linked to attempts to control other key infectious diseases (e.g., smallpox, cholera, leprosy, tuberculosis, and syphilis).

In many ways, our modern view of disease as a tangible and worldly "thing" that disrupts a naturally healthy body – and creates social problems – grows out of the upheavals linked to epidemics. Many things have obviously contributed to a secularized view of humanity, nature, and disease. The effects of epidemics on attitudes toward disease, health, and mortality are factors that help set the conditions for a physical approach to the self and its "scientific" investigation. The growth of hospitals as settings for care and the consolidation of the professions of surgery, medicine, and pharmacy are developments linked to a growing socialized and secular view of disease. All of these developments come to play increasing roles in the organization of the social system of medicine of Western states.

It is not possible to enumerate the different ways in which the structure and way of life in modern society have contributed to additional kinds of medical problems. Many types of chronic diseases, for example, are seen as produced by or endemic in contemporary states. Thus, a great deal of research on the "type A" behavior pattern has led to a specific formulation of human-environment factors in hypertension and cardiovascular disease. Certain cultural conditions (e.g., competitive challenges, deadlines) appear to combine with certain susceptible individuals (type A, which one should view as more typically "formed" under certain cultural conditions) to produce specific physiologic response (e.g., excess sympathetic responses, reduced blood-clotting time), which, if repeated sufficiently often, cause permanent damage to the cardiovascular system (Eyer, 1975). In essence, one could say that adverse cultural conditions can lead to permanent maladaptive nervous system responses; the "fixing" of these is associated with increased levels of morbidity and mortality. Similar formulations could be developed about other so-called chronic diseases and also about allied medical conditions (e.g., obesity, lung cancer, drug abuse), all of which can be judged as conditioned by the way of life or culture of modern civilization (Boyden, 1970).

In earlier historical eras, state interventions in public health have affected transportation of people and merchandise, led to the quarantine of suspected patients and to the fumigation of their belongings, and resulted in the imposition of medical care and hygienic practices regarding sanitation and food intake (Cartwright,

1977; Cipolla, 1973). In contemporary times, infectious diseases are much less burdensome and problems such as cardiovascular disease and cancer loom as significant. Given these types of diseases and the precedent of state intervention in public health, a logical outcome would appear to be campaigns against smoking and drinking, the promulgation of healthy diets and regular exercise, and, recently, the encouragement of "correct" principles of social and family relations, principles derived from government-supported research into the causes of medical problems. All of these "treatments" appear to be evolving into social directives aimed at the posited causes of disease that are predicated on our theory of illness. The ethical implications of these policies can be contested, but that they appear to flow out of our evolving system of medicine and create dilemmas seems very clear.

CHALLENGES POSED TO THE CONTEMPORARY THEORY OF ILLNESS

I have emphasized that in a basic sense the type of society and its mode of linkage to the physical environment — one can say, the culture-nature relationship — are what condition (in certain respects, determine) the kinds of medical problems that exist in a society. It is the set of medical problems that exist in a society that constitute the target of the society's theory of illness and medical care system. The latter phenomena, which one may term the cultural and sociological aspects of medicine, are what in turn condition (in certain respects, determine) how these problems are construed and handled. An emphasis on culture and ecology is necessary if one intends to study disease-illness and social approaches to disease-illness from a comparative and evolutionary standpoint. This way of viewing medical phenomena is consistent with tenets of cultural materialism (Harris, 1979). An understanding of the idea of medicalization seems incomplete if evolutionary concerns are excluded.

The historical and evolutionary trend outlined previously covers a time segment during which, one could say, humans came to acquire progressively greater control of nature and also came progressively to incorporate nature into human frames of purpose and action. Indeed, the idea of "environment" has come to include the social as well as the physical, both of which are partly created and shaped by people. The change in the way humans and social groups now relate to nature is described by Bennett (1979) as involving an "ecological transition." This transition has included changes in technology (e.g., use of ever-larger quantities of energy), history-sociology (e.g., evolution of nations, the proliferation of status hierarchies), ecology (e.g., breakdown of local self-sufficiency), economics (e.g., industrialization, commerce), and philosophy (e.g., changes in the image that humans have of themselves as active and productive beings).

The ecological transition, when carried over into the contemporary era, is associated with an increased level of certain diseases and also has led to what is often described as a medicalization of human concerns. One graphic example of this is provided by "problems" such as baldness, facial wrinkles, cosmetically undesirable physical traits, the wish to avoid pregnancy, and personal worry — demoralization about one's accomplishments or status. For each of these problems we could be said to have a medical technology of care consisting, for example, of plastic surgery, contraceptives, and psychotherapy. The conditions listed above can be judged as "medical problems" in the trivial sense that physicians and the prevailing system of medicine have evolved the respective technologies for treatment. In a less trivial sense, however, these conditions are sometimes justified as medical or as illnesses because they can lead to an impairment in (psychological) well-being and (social) functioning. That these concerns are equated with illnesses seems counterintuitive and supportive of the claim that medicalization is taking place in contemporary societies. How is one to understand problems such as the above, and how are the dilemmas they pose to be handled?

Personal concerns and worries are universal, and in all types of societies certain individuals are plagued by them. Unfortunately, the kinds of personal concerns and worries that members of different types of society have is a topic that has not often been studied directly in anthropology, much less so the range of private concerns. In a broad sense, such concerns can be said to be shaped by the form of the culture-nature interaction that exists at the time. It would seem that a study of the cultural ecology would include topics centering on subsistence and group integrity: for example, the level of resources in the immediate local environment, the quality of relations with outside groups, and the intentions and motivations of co-members, preternatural agents, and ancestors. One assumes that to this inventory could be added concerns involving personal health and normality, health of living relatives, and status of social relations in the group. Each type and/or level of society can be viewed as generating a matrix of personal concerns that are conditioned by the form of its culture-nature interaction. A reading of ethnographical literature quickly convinces one that, in small-scale societies, actual episodes of illness are, in a symbolic sense, made up of many such personal concerns and worries (Fabrega, 1974). In other words, personal worries and concerns of everyday life are integral to the theory of illness of the society and serve as actual explanations of illness episodes. Indeed, one could say that a small-scale society's theory of illness partially chronicles the types of concerns and worries of the members in it. A review of the early social history of Western and Eastern civilizations would no doubt reveal inventories of personal concerns and worries not less conditioned by the form of the prevailing culture-nature interaction and no less overlapping with symbolizations and health and illness.

In contemporary medicine, we tend to no longer use the language of personal concerns when we explain illness. Instead, we use the language of physiology and chemistry — and in some instances of "stressors" or "emotional conflicts." The latter terminology can be looked at as a way of impersonalizing and, from a social standpoint, decontextualizing a medical problem. In speaking about illness with this type of language we appear to separate the "medical" from the "social" or "psychological."

The technical language of biomedicine obscures the fact that what people worry about are the consequences of physical states of disease, including pain, disability, and interferences in psychosocial functioning. Facial wrinkles and other socially disvalued physical markers are not diseases, but concern and worry over them is "natural" given that people now live longer and, moreover, seem oriented toward youth, physical attractiveness, and materialistic values. Fears of pregnancy and/or feelings of demoralization or dissatisfaction (the "treatment" of which is contraceptives and psychotherapy) are also not diseases in the modern sense, but they are concerns and worries of the type that, from a comparative point of view, seem to have repeatedly been medicalized in one way or another. Should these examples appear trivial, one could add others such as anorexia nervosa, "cardiac neurosis," and cancer phobias, that is, types of personal concerns and worries that can be accompanied by crippling physiological symptoms and that seem conditioned by the symbolic environment that contemporary civilization is producing. In other words, personal concerns and worries are outgrowths of the cultural standards, values, and emphases that exist in a society and can be seen as produced in much the way diseases are produced. The concerns and worries singled out here grow out of the contemporary culture-nature interaction, an interaction that produces new life-styles, new knowledge about the body, and new perspectives about the self.

One who reduces medical problems to physical factors concentrates on genes, biochemistry, physiology, and disease entities and examines how these are affected by the culture-nature interaction that prevails in the society in question. Symbolizations about personal concerns, including those of illness, are likely to be judged as incidental "surface phenomena," far removed from the substantive aspects of disease. Importance may be granted to personal concerns should they lead to practices that are deleterious to physical health status or should they occasion enough "emotional disturbance" so as to render an individual more prone or vulnerable to clearly specified disease processes. In either event, it is clear that a great deal of parsimony and power are gained when medical problems are reduced to a strict biomedical level, for then traditional biological parameters of survival and reproduction are invoked as integral to disease accounting (Fabrega, 1979). Anchoring medical problems to biomedical facts such as these might allow one to more easily make social decisions and policy recommendations. A limitation of the reductionist's program, however, is that suffering, functioning, and level and quality of adaptation, phenomena intrinsic to what illness means in a general anthropological frame of reference, are excluded.

In contrast to the above, one who emphasizes the interconnections between biological, psychological, and social factors will judge individuals holistically, resist body-mind partitioning, and describe a medical problem or illness as something rooted in and expressed by social adaptation and function (Engel, 1977). To such an individual, personal concerns and worries are important, for they not only register the meanings of an adaptive failure or illness but also partially account for it. In resisting the biomedical reductionist stance, those who argue for the importance of a psychosocial posture point to the "systems view of man" and see in the principle of psychosomatic mediation a device that explains how personal concerns can link to and disturb bodily systems and why adaptation and maladaptation or illness are characterizations about whole persons. A limitation of the holist's program is the possible inclusion as legitimate medical problems personal concerns and worries that can raise the question of medicalization. In summary, it would seem that both types of analysts (i.e., those guided by strict biomedical versus those who embrace the psychosocial) would judge personal concerns and worries as influential in the kinds of medical problems that are prevalent in a society but would place altogether different degrees of emphasis on them.

CONCLUSIONS

The medical system of a society may be described as the composite of traditions, beliefs, practices, and institutions for dealing with illness that is a condition of the whole individual and that has a behavioral structure of some sort. In small-scale societies, medical systems are not clearly differentiated from other "systems" of the society — for example, the religious or political. What this means is that in those societies illness is understood and dealt with in terms of ideas and practices that also have religious and political overtones. Given the mode of functioning of such societies, one could claim that what from our standpoint are medical phenomena, in small-scale societies are socialized (or politicized) and, conversely, that social problems are medicalized. Clearly, this claim could not be made by the people themselves, since the meaning of "medical" is precisely what they judge and do about illness.

A striking feature of our modern and evolved medical system is its relative independence from other social systems. The processes of diagnosis and treatment of illness in modern societies constitute enterprises that involve knowledge and practices that have, relatively speaking, fewer immediate religious and political overtones. The relative independence of our medical system from that of other social systems can be seen as one consequence of the processes of modernization, the growth of science, and, generally, secularization. Nevertheless, very often in modern societies phenomena that we judge as social, such as certain types of deviances, or personal, such as worries and preoccupations about cancer or facial wrinkles, are judged and handled as though they were medical. From a strict bio-medical standpoint, one could claim that, in modern societies, psychosocial phenomena are medicalized. From a general anthropological point of view, however, it is difficult to sustain this claim, since the meaning of "medical" varies greatly.

The idea of medicalization is often used in a historical and evolutionary sense, but its value here can be questioned. At any time when we examine how a society is viewing and handling illness, we are examining a problem that in a concrete sense is conditioned by its ecology, history, sociology, and culture and, moreover, is a problem that in an analytical sense is construed in terms of symbols and conventions that grow out of, and are based on, the same ecological, historical, sociological, and cultural influences. Given this interconnection between illness prevalence and illness symbolization — more generally, culture, social perspectives, and ecology — we are being highly ethnocentric when we say that certain societies medicalize social happenings more than others or, conversely, that some societies differentially "socialize" (or politicize or religiously color) medical happenings. In brief, approaches to illness and approaches to other problems and concerns need to be seen in the same cultural context. What a society terms "medical" grows out of a distinctive culture-ecology context and is in certain respects just as social or conventional as anything else. It is somewhat ethnocentric to reason as though our current distinctions and ideologies are correct and universal or as though earlier societies operated with misguided ones.

The idea of medicalization, when used by contemporary social critics, seems to imply several things. One of these is that phenomena so inherently physical-bodily and personal (i.e., involving disease) should not be dealt with as social or psychological; another is, conversely, that phenomena that are psychological or social are really not medical since they are not the outcome of an underlying disease. A reductionist rhetoric about medical problems overlooks the conventional character of illness. Such rhetoric also obscures the important analytical distinction that exists between illness and disease and the many dilemmas that grow out of our evolving theory of illness that seems based on the distinction. These dilemmas require that a rational scientific theory of illness be developed as a basis for guiding social policy and action.

REFERENCES

Bennett, J. 1979. *The Ecological Transition.* New York: Random House.

Boyden, S. V., ed. 1970. *The Impact of Civilization on the Biology of Man.* Toronto: University of Toronto Press.

Cartwright, F. F. 1977. *Social History of Medicine.* New York: Longman.

Cipolla, C. 1973. *Christofano and the Plague: A Study of the History of Public Health in the Age of Galileo.* Berkeley: University of California Press.

Engel, G. L. 1977. The Need for a New Medical Model: A Challenge for Biomedicine. *Science* 196:129-36.

Eyer, J. 1975. Hypertension as a Disease of Modern Society. *Int. J. Health Serv.* 5:539-58.

Fabrega, H., Jr. 1974. *Disease and Social Behavior: An Interdisciplinary Perspective.* Cambridge, Mass.: M.I.T. Press.

———. 1975. The Need for an Ethnomedicine Science. *Science* 189:969-75.

———. 1979. The Scientific Usefulness of the Idea of Illness. *Perspect. Biol. Med.* 22:545-58.

———. Elementary Systems of Medicine. *Cult. Med. Psychiatry*, in press.

Fabrega, H., and Silver, D. 1973. *Illness and Shamanistic Curing in Zinacantan.* Stanford, Calif.: Stanford University Press.

Harris, M. 1979. *Cultural Materialism.* New York: Random House.

Illich, I. 1976. *Medical Nemesis: The Expropriation of Health.* New York: Pantheon.

Lasch, C. 1977. *Haven in a Heartless World: The Family Beseiged.* New York: Basic.

3

ON MEDICALIZATION AND THE TRIUMPH OF THE THERAPEUTIC

Christopher Lasch

The historical process of medicalization is best understood, in the West at least, as the "triumph of the therapeutic," as Rieff (1966) calls it. The spiritual center of our society, according to Rieff, has shifted from the church to the statehouse and, in our own time, to the hospital. The decline of religion, followed by the decline of the political culture that briefly took its place in the nineteenth century, has left Western man destitute of transcendent goals. Now what is searched for is neither salvation nor the creation of the good society on earth but a sense of health and well-being. The categories of sin and crime have given way to sickness, a form of deviance amenable to therapeutic intervention. Religious and civil forms of authority have yielded to therapeutic authority and political and economic man to psychological man, who seeks no higher end, in Rieff's formulation, than to beguile the time.

Cross-cultural approaches to the study of medicalization shed little light on medicalization in the West, except by contrast. In primitive societies, most phases of life fall under priestly authority. Because religion in such societies retains so many characteristics of magic, religion and medicine are not clearly distinguished. The merging of priestly and medical authority makes it possible, in turn, for tribal cultures undergoing Westernization selectively to absorb modern medical practice while preserving much of the immemorial folk medicine of their ancestors. The coexistence of folk medicine with Western medicine, side by side, helps to distinguish such societies from our own. In the West, scientific technology has eroded popular traditions of healing and self-help, replaced popular culture with a technological and therapeutic culture, and made people increasingly dependent on scientific experts not merely for the satisfaction of their needs but for the very definition of their needs.

Modern therapeutic authority depends for its effectiveness on the cooperation of the patient. The condition of treatment is that the patient acknowledge a sickness (revealed in aberrant behavior that might otherwise be attributed to malingering, selfishness, or some other moral failing), acknowledge the therapist's professional qualifications for treating it, and cooperate with the regimen that is prescribed. A therapeutic culture cannot be imposed on an unwilling population. Since modern professionals (unlike those who wield civil or religious authority) have no sanction, as Freidson (1970) has pointed out, except the client's need of their services, a major part of medical practice has consisted of attempts to create and sustain a demand for medical services. The medical education of the public presupposes a population already disposed to accept scientific explanations of phenomena — causal thinking as opposed to magical thinking. In a culture still dominated by magical thinking, modern medicine is absorbed into the existing structures of magic, instead of presenting itself as a rival order of explanation that challenges and undermines older systems of thought.

Medicalization in the West has to be seen, then, as a specific configuration — the principal features of which I shall outline in a moment — arising out of a specific historical development. Consider the transformation of crime into sickness. The substitution of political authority for priestly authority gave rise, in the eighteenth century, to the classical liberal theory of criminology, according to which crime is punished not to protect the community of believers (as in the Inquisition) or even to protect a state that itself identifies its interests with the church and claims divine origin, but to protect individuals from actions that infringe on their natural, self-evident rights. Under liberal theory and practice, as Kittrie puts in it *The Right To Be Different* (1971, p. 20), "the criminal is punished because he is a man whose free will makes him responsible for his acts; if his acts infringe upon the rights of others, he should pay."

In the nineteenth century, this rationalistic, utilitarian approach to the problem of crime gave way to an allegedly scientific, deterministic way of thinking, in which crime is the product of bad social conditions. The new criminology founded on this premise, and on an analogy with the public health movement, sought not to punish crime but to prevent it and not to treat the symptoms of social disorder but to remove their cause. Modern criminology pleads for understanding of criminals on the grounds that they bear no responsibility for their actions; at the same time, however, it has replaced criminal sanctions with a more subtle and pervasive system of social controls, which tries to enlist the cooperation of the "patients" in their own "cure." Reformation and rehabilitation replace retribution as the goals of criminal jurisprudence. In many ways an advance on earlier practice, the advent of medical jurisprudence or "psychiatric justice" (Szasz, 1965) nevertheless undermines individual rights and makes it more difficult for people accused of crimes to defend themselves against the state.

Eighteenth and early nineteenth century liberalism assumed that the pursuit of self-interest is the principal determinant of human conduct, hence the need for laws to protect the weak against the strong. Twentieth century humanitarians believe, on the other hand, that people act from irrational motives, that they are in addition the products of culture (not free will), and that therefore they cannot always be held responsible for their actions. Formerly the court regarded the actions of adults as deliberate and calculating – this being one of the ways in which they presumably differed from the actions of minors. Today the courts accept the psychiatric view that "man is an integrated personality," as Bazelon (1954) once put it, "and that reason is only one element in that personality, not the sole determinant of his conduct." On these grounds, Bazelon overturned an old rule under which the courts allowed a plea of insanity only if the defendant showed no ability to distinguish between right and wrong. He argued instead that an accused person is not criminally responsible if the unlawful act was the product of mental disease or mental defect.

With these historical examples in mind, we can say that medicalization implies a number of interrelated changes peculiar to the West. It implies, first of all, an expansion of professional control at the expense of older traditions of healing (e.g., herbal medicine, home remedies, midwifery).

Second, it implies an expansion of the conditions labeled as sickness and requiring medical "treatment," as opposed to religious, civil, or other intervention.

Third, it redefines as therapeutic relationships, doctor-patient relationships, relationships that were formerly adversarial. Increasingly, citizens confront the state not as an adversary, with a clear understanding of the rights of both parties, but as a source of friendly medical assistance. This change reduces citizens to consumers of professional services, and it makes it more difficult for them to resist coercion when it comes in the guise of help.

Fourth, medicalization presupposes a new model of human behavior, a new model of personality that stresses the primacy of irrational impulse and/or culturally determined patterns of response, as opposed to free choice, rational calculation, and enlightened self-interest.

Finally, medicalization requires the internalization of medical authority in the population as a whole — the spread of a new way of thinking about freedom and responsibility: a culture of the therapeutic.

The net result of this process is to weaken the sense of moral responsibility and also the capacity for self-help. Therapeutic modes of thought and practice exempt their object, the patients, from critical judgment and relieve them of moral responsibility. Sickness by definition represents an invasion of patients by forces outside their control, at least outside their conscious control, and the patients' realistic recognition of the limits of their own responsibility — their acceptance of their diseased and helpless condition — constitutes the first step toward recovery (or permanent invalidism, as the case may be). Therapy labels as sickness what might otherwise be judged as weak or wilful actions. It thus equips patients to fight (or become resigned to) their disease, instead of irrationally finding fault with themselves. Inappropriately extended beyond the consulting room, however, therapeutic morality encourages a permanent atrophy of the moral sense. There is a close connection, in turn, between the erosion of moral responsibility and the waning of the capacity for self-help — in the categories used by Seeley, between the elimination of culpability and the elimination of competence. "What says 'you are not guilty' says also 'you cannot help yourself'" (Seeley, 1967, p. 90). Therapy legitimates deviance as sickness, but it simultaneously pronounces patients as unfit to manage their own lives and delivers them into the hands of a specialist. As therapeutic points of view and practice gain general acceptance, more and more people find themselves disqualified, in effect, from the performance of adult roles and responsibilities and become dependent on some form of medical authority.

Having described the consequences of medicalization in a rather sinister light, I should add that I do not regard medicalization as a conspiracy of the "helping professions." Those who designed the therapeutic state (if we can even speak of it as the product of design) saw it not as an agency of repression but as an agency of social improvement and personal liberation. It is unfortunate that modern professionalism took shape at a time when widespread fears of social disorder, class conflict, violence, and crime predisposed the propertied classes, and many professionals themselves, to seize on the new professionalism as an instrument of social control. In the United States and western Europe, the period roughly from 1848 to 1914 was a period of rapid change and social upheaval, in which popular movements challenged the ascendancy of property and called up the specter of a revolutionary overthrow of established institutions. The transition from classical liberalism to twentieth century progressivism reflected these fears and the search for new principles of order and social cohesion. The development of modern professionalism, in which a medical model of human behavior was generalized into a program of social improvement and social engineering, was deeply colored by the historical context in which it took place — by the prevailing social anxieties of the time. Under these conditions, the science or would-be science of social pathology commended itself as the answer to the problem of social disorder — as a nonrevolutionary solution to the tensions and strains of the advanced industrial order. Revisionist historians of professionalization, by stressing the self-aggrandizing ambitions of the professions themselves, have missed the larger picture and presented a conspiratorial interpretation of changes that came about for complicated reasons and cannot be disentangled, moreover, from the genuine progress of human understanding, compassion, and sensitivity to suffering.

REFERENCES

Bazelon, D. L. 1954. Opinion in *Durham v. U.S.* (1954), quoted in *Psychiatry* 17:286, 297.

Freidson, E. 1970. *Professional Dominance: The Social Structure of Medical Care*. New York: Atherton.

Kittrie, N. N. 1971. *The Right To Be Different*. Baltimore: Johns Hopkins University Press.

Rieff, P. 1966. *The Triumph of the Therapeutic*. New York: Harper & Row.

Seeley, J. R. 1967. Parents — The Last Proletariat. In *The Americanization of the Unconscious*, ed. J. R. Seeley. New York: International Science Press.

Szasz, T. S. 1965. *Psychiatric Justice*. New York: Macmillan.

4

MEDICALIZATION AND THE CLINICAL PRAXIS OF MEDICAL SYSTEMS

Arthur Kleinman

The views presented thus far seem split between the medical historian asserting "medicalization" is a fairly recent phenomenon in the West that is utterly distinct from indigenous medical systems in non-Western societies and the medical anthropologists who retort that in cross-cultural perspective medicalization is neither unique to the West nor interpretable solely from the standpoint of recent Western sociohistorical change.

While recognizing that the nature of medicalization in twentieth century America and Europe undoubtedly is distinctive, I side with anthropology. Medical systems are cultural systems in all societies. As a result, they possess universal clinical structures and functions, albeit these disclose considerable cross-cultural variation. Medicalization needs to be interpreted, then, in terms of culturally constituted clinical categories and praxis. From the standpoint of medicine defined as a cultural system, medicalization is not uniquely Western, although the form medicalization has assumed in the contemporary West is specific to that historical and cultural context.

HEALTH CARE SYSTEM

In prior work I have described in detail a model of medical systems (which I have referred to as health care systems) in society that is applicable across both historical and cultural boundaries (Kleinman, 1980). The model defines medical systems as cultural systems in which sickness is articulated as a symbolic form of social life and therapy is applied within specific social structural sectors that contain distinctive beliefs, norms, social roles, and relationships. In contemporary Western and non-Western societies, three sectors (or arenas) of care can be described; (1) professional (both Western and indigenous therapeutic professions), (2) folk (nonprofessionalized indigenous specialists), and (3) popular (i.e., family, social network, community) sectors.

Medical systems and their sectors can be described as interconnected systems of meanings, norms, and power. Within these cultural systems sickness is experienced, explained, and treated in terms of particular participants' explanatory models of sickness, norms governing patient and practitioner behavior, and differences in power. These features of medical systems differ for their different sectors so that the same individual with the same sickness crossing the boundaries between sectors encounters often distinctive clinical realities (i.e., socially constructed forms of clinical communication and practice).

Medical systems perform six universal clinical tasks:

1. The cultural construction of socially learned and sanctioned *illness* experience and behavior out of biologically determined *disease*

2. The cultural construction of strategies and evaluative criteria to guide choices among alternative health care practices and practitioners and to evaluate the process and, most importantly, the outcome (efficacy) of clinical care

3. The cognitive and communicative processes involved in the management of sickness, including labeling, classifying, and providing personally and socially meaningful explanations

4. Healing activities *per se*, including all types of therapeutic interventions, from diet, drugs, and surgery to psychotherapy, supportive care, and healing rituals

5. Deliberate and nondeliberate health enhancing (largely preventive) and health lowering (sickness producing) behaviors

6. The management of a range of therapeutic outcomes, including cure, treatment failure, recurrence, chronic illness, impairment, and death.

Different medical systems and sectors may be more involved with a particular clinical function than others, and the ways these core clinical tasks are performed also will reflect cultural, historicopolitical, economic, and ecological determinants. Furthermore, as medical systems change, so do their ways of performing clinical work.

MEDICALIZATION AS A CULTURAL PHENOMENON

First, medical systems in different societies or in different historical periods differ in what is and is not labeled as sickness or as medically-relevant aspects of social life. They also can and frequently do differ with respect to the types and number of health problems that are managed in the different sectors or subsectors. Power differentials between sectors and subsectors also obviously are different. Personal and group interests, control and distribution of scarce resources and many other aspects of medical systems are revealed by cross-cultural research to vary, sometimes markedly. For example, it has been noted by many investigators (cf. Kleinman, 1979) that personal and group involvement with health and health care concerns is greater in Chinese communities than in Northern European and American ones. That is to say, the importance and cultural space of medical systems differ across cultures and in different historical times. Moreover, within China's medical system, Unschuld (1979) argues that conflict over control of scarce resources among competing medical groups has historically included ethical debates that provide ideological sanctioning for relative advantage of one medical group vis-à-vis the others. This is, in essence, a struggle over control of medicalization.

From this perspective, medicalization is a much more complex process than it is usually regarded. Certain traditional societies, for example, rely on medical systems as their chief and sometimes their only means of social control (Cawte, 1974). Compared with these usually small-scale preliterate societies, what we have been calling medicalization in the contemporary West is less total and extreme. Use of the medical system as an institution of social control is ubiquitous, so much so that social control can be added to our list of core functions. Comparative descriptions of the historical development of medical systems along with other social systems with respect to modernization, Westernization, and indigenizations have only recently been initiated (Kleinman et al., 1975; Leslie, 1976), and we still await a synthesis that will inform us of cross-cultural similarities and differences in the way life problems and institutions are medicalized or demedicalized.

A second insight gained from the model of the medical system as a cultural system is recognition that taxonomic or institutional medicalization can involve the entire system or one of its sectors or subsectors. For example, much of the current concern with medicalization in the West clearly centers on the professional sector and especially on the biomedical subsector of medical systems. Indeed, some commentators have argued that professional medicalization occurs at the expense of the other sectors, so that the popular and folk sectors reciprocally demedicalize. Conversely, other commentators contest that medicalization in our society involves all three sectors, although the professional sector predominates.

Part of the problem is definitional. By medicalization do we refer to meanings, norms, or power, or all of these features of cultural systems? In much of the world, for instance, illness episodes are treated solely in the popular sector, most usually in its family subsector (Kleinman, 1980). That means that in most medical systems (traditional and modern) the popular sector is the chief source of health care. When examining professional medicalization, we should simultaneously look at changes in the popular sector. This interrelationship can be examined with regard to changes in status, access to and control over limited resources (knowledge as well as material resources), official legitimation, and sanctioned cultural idioms for articulating distress (e.g., somatic, psychological, moral, cosmological). Contemporary medicalization in the West, for example, has involved biomedicalization and psychologization of problems previously defined as legal, moral, or religious. And this process has involved all three sectors of the medical system. Westernization of third world societies has frequently included biomedicalization and psychologization as well. These have been part and parcel of the social development processes of urbanization, bureaucratization, and professionalization. However, these processes may displace an earlier form of medicalization in which, as in Taiwan, problems are defined in cosmological or naturalistic idioms because the system of folk religion and the system of traditional Chinese medicine were the predominant therapeutic (or in broader terms, social coping) approaches. Ferguson (1981) shows that in El Salvador, and in other Latin American societies, medicalization is principally on behalf of commercial pharmaceutical interests (local pharmacies' practices are economically dominated by international pharmaceutical firms and their local surrogates, and these practices in turn strongly influence popular and even folk drug use). Ferguson's findings highlight that substantial and frequently damaging medicalization may occur without professional medical control as a result of the commercial pharmaceutical professional subsector and the sociopolitical interests it serves both domestically and worldwide. This is an important correction to the professional paranoia of Illich and his epigones, who see medicalization as the sin of doctors. In many societies, legislators, local bureaucrats, pharmacists, social workers, medical journalists and television commentators, and business interests (e.g., drug companies, profit-making laboratories) are among the chief sources of medicalization.

Medicalization of life problems may be regarded from a cultural perspective as an important coping strategy. Managing stress and social problems has been available to cultural systems in different therapeutic forms — shamanism, traditional medicine, biomedicine, and self-care. It simply is wrongheaded to regard it as monolithic or necessarily maladaptive. Indeed the cross-cultural literature suggests that it has had adaptive as well as maladaptive effects. In other work I have developed this argument in detail (Kleinman, 1980); here I wish only to underline the universal aspects of medicalization as a complement to its culture-specific features. Cross-cultural comparisons teach us to be cautious that our usage of the term "medicalization" be neither ethnocentric nor profession centered as a result of the implicit cultural bias of our society's clinical categories. Medicalization is a most appropriate subject for comparative cross-cultural and historical empirical studies of medical systems. Removed from the cultural context of medical systems, the concept of medicalization is all too easily misinterpreted and abused for ideological purposes, not the least of which is a reverse ethnocentrism and historical romanticism that seeks to criticize, albeit with redistributive justice, the excesses of the contemporary health professions and the extratherapeutic (and often repugnant) social functions of our clinical categories and praxis. While I personally share many of these criticisms, I think it is a serious error to simplify and confuse the critique of health and medicine in contemporary society by calling it medicalization. Instead of encouraging this fallacy of misplaced concreteness, we need to refine our use of this term and understand medicalization as a complex, multisided cultural and social process. Here empirical studies are crucial. For if, as Bateson (1979) insists, explanation is the mapping of description onto tautology, it is essential that we understand medicalization as a most powerful and little-examined contemporary cultural tautology that is best illuminated by actual, detailed ethnographic case studies and systematic rigorous cross-cultural comparisons.

But my point is also that, while social scientists should exercise restraint in applying the label "medicalization," physicians and health planners should be taught about medicalization as a clinical heuristic to sensitize them to its potentially dangerous consequences and to aid them to use restraint in accepting their roles as society's agents of medicalization. The social science critique of the negative medicalizing effects of the community mental health ideology, for example, has forced psychiatrists and mental health professionals generally to be more restrained about the application of clinical categories to social problems and to be more aware of the limits of the therapeutic. But this important clinical heuristic effect will be rapidly undermined if medicalization is not operationalized as a discrete, data-based, clinically applicable concept but instead is abused as an ideological weapon. Medicalization is too important a concept to be so misused.

Overstatement of biomedical critiques is an occupational hazard of social scientists in medicine for at least two well-known reasons: (1) the marginal status of and inattention to social science in the health field often encourages exaggeration and invective as a defense against isolation and helplessness and (2) practical clinical application of social science concepts is viewed negatively by some social scientists because it potentially can increase medicalization by better arming clinicians to be more effective in conceptualizing and managing psychosocial problems. Both positions are dangerous.

Social scientists can and indeed have exerted important influences in clinical care. They have done so by operationalizing concepts such as sick role and illness behavior so that they can be practically taught and applied in everyday patient care. Treating medicalization in the same fashion is a responsibility of the clinical social scientist. Similarly, social scientists working with health planners can be effective in translating medicalization in terms that can positively influence the planning of health services. Of course, from the wider medical system perspective, social science's ideological struggle to redefine clinical reality with biomedicine, in which the term "medicalization" increasingly looms large, also is needed to bring about change in medical systems. But such conflict is clearly benefited by a more discriminating cross-cultural understanding of medicalization — hence my plea that medicalization be treated as a serious source of hypotheses for cross-cultural and historical empirical studies that yield data that feed back to make this concept more suitable for clinical and public health applications. Otherwise, like some other potentially useful social science concepts, this term will be trivialized and rendered irrelevant.

In 1981 in the United States not the least of the aspects of the social process that require assessment is the systematic undermining of the public subsector of the professional sector of health care systems by the ruling political forces in favor of commercial interests that threaten to demedicalize the former while extending the power and control of the latter. That is to say, we in America are in the midst of a major alteration in the nature and consequences of medicalization that makes the very term seem somewhat obsolete and peripheral to the core developments around us. Perhaps we have arrived at the limits of medicalization as a useful window on developments in our own society, although it may still be of use in studies of developing societies. In any event the term has become so polysemic that we require not only differentiation and focus on demedicalization but also a whole new set of concepts to describe what is now taking place in the West.

REFERENCES

Bateson, G. 1979. *Mind and Nature.* New York: Dutton.

Cawte, J. E. 1974. *Medicine Is the Law: Studies in Psychiatric Anthropology of Australian Tribal Societies.* Honolulu: University of Hawaii Press.

Ferguson, A. E. 1981. Commercial Pharmaceutical Medicine and Medicalization: A Case Study from El Salvador. *Culture Med. Psychiatry* 5:105-34.

Kleinman, A. 1980. *Patients and Healers in the Context of Culture: An Exploration of the Borderland between Anthropology, Medicine, and Psychiatry.* Berkeley: University of California Press.

Kleinman, A., et al., eds. 1975. *Medicine in Chinese Cultures.* Washington, D.C.: The Fogarty International Center, National Institutes of Health.

Leslie, C., ed. 1976. *Asian Medical Systems*. Berkeley: University of California Press.

Unschuld, P. 1979. *Medical Ethics in Imperial China*. Berkeley: University of California Press.

PART II

Becoming an Illness: The Couvade Example

A central conceptual problem in any debate about uses and abuses of medicine or about medicalization relates to the nature of medical problems and their solutions. We include this section on the couvade phenomenon both because of its intrinsic interest and because it casts fresh light on our views of the nature of illness and of how people and practitioners organize themselves in relation to it.

Couvade is the occurrence of pregnancy-like phenomena in the mates of expectant women. Used by anthropologists, it refers to male rituals related to pregnancy or birth. Used clinically, it refers to the occurrence of pregnancy related signs or symptoms in the mate of a pregnant woman.

Becoming an illness begins with an in-depth look at the organization of a small society in New Guinea concerning pregnancy and birth. In Chapter 5, Poole illustrates the rich interactions between the physical event of pregnancy and the complex belief system of the Bimin-Kuskusmin. The men in this society experience multiple life changes, notably changes in dwelling, diet, and interpersonal relations during their mate's pregnancy. Part of this process is the occurrence of physical symptoms that are readily recognized by society as relating to pregnancy. Because the tribe notes that the Western healers in a nearby clinic do not recognize these relationships, they feel Western care cannot be effective. Hence, they shun the Western clinic in this situation because it lacks sufficient diagnostic categories. Poole concludes that under these conditions, Western care *under*medicalizes by failing to adequately deal with the social context of illness phenomena.

In Rochester, New York, a related albeit distinct phenomenon occurs. Lipkin and Lamb show in Chapter 6, that 22.5 percent of men seek care for symptoms that fit the criteria for couvade condition during their mate's pregnancy. These men, in contrast to the Bimin-Kuskusmin, do not recognize this connection nor do their physicians. They have three times the expected number of medical visits, twice the expected number of prescriptions, and many tests and procedures they might not have needed had this phenomenon been recognized. The authors discuss the presentation and possible mechanism of this phenomenon in their sample. They imply that the failure to recognize social or psychological causes of problems may lead to an overly narrow, biomedically oriented approach to explanation, diagnosis, and treatment, which may be inappropriate, expensive, and hazardous.

Serendipitously, Gabriel, in the same city, was interviewing fathers-to-be about their new role. Her results in Chapter 7 reinforce the findings of Lipkin and Lamb and show that this phenomenon has broader manifestations beyond their conservative set of symptoms. Gabriel reports, anecdotally, that change of behavior of fathers-to-be in relation to diet is common and may serve several social purposes, including bringing their new status to the attention of others, protecting them against ill health, and serving as a "rite of passage."

In Chapter 8, Harper takes a precise sociological analysis as his starting point. He defines "medicalization" as a term to describe the social process of "making medical" and notes that it can be used both descriptively and normatively and can be judged correct or incorrect or good or bad, depending on the criteria of the judges. He notes that signification processes include labeling and argues that medical labeling can, like criminal labeling, alter the behavior of those who give the label and those who receive it. After questioning whether couvade represents "negative" labeling, in which the application of the label creates the named conditions, he decides it does not. Instead, he invokes mental mechanisms, which he feels intervene between a wife's pregnancy and a man's symptoms.

Lipkin, then, attempts an iteration and analysis of the sequence of events that occur in the typical case of Western couvade. He notes that each of the many steps are socially effected and can lead to psychological, social, and physical effects. He then specifies at least three distinct mechanisms for couvade. The first is the translation of emotional events into body language and the use of the body language as metacommunication. The second is the occurrence of minor bodily changes, also interpretable as language, which lead in turn to symptoms. The third is the occurrence of psychophysiological changes that lead to pathological alterations, in this case hemor-rhoidal bleeding. Lipkin uses this analysis to conclude that a proper model of illness includes recognition of the existence of multiple causal chains in the creation, experience, and sustaining of illness and shows some of the problems caused by failure to include suffici-ent factors in the understanding of presented symptoms. These include failure to detect common phenomena, such as couvade. They include excessive and inappropriate search in one level, usually the physical, with unnecessary expense and harm. He argues that if a causal link is omitted in clinical thinking its omission will go undetected and lead to the insularity of view that presently charac-terizes the dominant biomedical paradigms. Lipkin concludes that the main issue is less that of medicalization or not, but rather that of the *appropriateness* of the models used in medicine. In general, too little psychological, social, and cultural information is used and too much physical information is sought.

5

COUVADE AND CLINIC IN A NEW GUINEA SOCIETY:
Birth Among the Bimin-Kuskusmin

Fitz John Porter Poole

> . . . birth is no unimportant event, and it is perfectly natural for both parents to do it.
>
> —— Marcel Mauss (quoted in Dumont, 1972, p. 10)

With increasing interest in problems of "medicalization" (see Fox, 1977; Illich, 1976), normal birth-related phenomena provide a popular example of what Sedgwick calls "the progressive annexation of not-illness into illness" (1973, p. 37). Birth is often cited as an instance in Western societies when biomedical labeling may preclude sensitivity to significant cultural, social, and psychological aspects of childbearing in gynecological-obstetrical practice.[1] In this essay, I examine selected aspects of birth events among the Bimin-Kuskusmin of the West Sepik interior of Papua New Guinea (see Poole, 1976a,b for general ethnographic background).[2] I emphasize *birth as a social process*, involving not only cultural constructions of birth events but also social management of childbearing by female midwives (Poole, 1981c) and close male and female kin. I focus on those adult males entering (or reentering) social parenthood whom Bimin-Kuskusmin call "pregnant fathers" (*arep aur kumun*). Such men are subject to elaborate ritual restrictions and, in the Bimin-Kuskusmin view, are variably vulnerable to stresses that are peculiar to the life-crisis of birth (see also Poole, 1981a).

In this regard, I explore three interrelated concerns: (1) the sociocultural significance of couvade ritual phenomena among Bimin-Kuskusmin;[3] (2) the significance of more variable psychophysiological couvade symptoms that are recognized, interpreted, and managed by Bimin-Kuskusmin in relation to traditional notions of birth-related stress and therapeutic adjustments in couvade ritual behavior;[4] and (3) the general refusal of Bimin-Kuskusmin to accept gynecological-obstetrical services at local Western clinics, from which they seek other kinds of medical assistance. I suggest that the Bimin-Kuskusmin view of Western belief and practice in regard to childbearing may be characterized as one of *under*medicalization, for Bimin-Kuskusmin tend to believe that Western clinical practice focuses exclusively on the dyad of mother and child as being the only people at risk in birth events. The Bimin-Kuskusmin view suggests that local clinics, because they do not appreciate the intricate sociocultural fabric and "embeddedness" of birth-related phenomena, do not intrude far enough into the *social process of birth* and, therefore, increase the already considerable risks of birth. To make sense of this perspective, the Bimin-Kuskusmin couvade (*men am aiyem ben* ["sacred womb rite"]) provides an illuminating ethnographical focus for analysis.

Despite much definitional controversy, the term "couvade" generally has been taken by anthropologists to refer to all patterned aspects of behavior (both overt and covert) associated with childbirth that involve the father giving up routine activities and taking on a variable range of behavioral prescriptions and proscriptions. As Rivière (1974) notes, however, analytical approaches to couvade have been shaped by historical shifts in anthropological interests and modes of interpretation (cf. Dawson, 1929; Frazer, 1910; Malinowski, 1927). Thus, although notions of some mystical connection between father and child have been widely recognized, interpretations of the phenomenon have been quite varied (cf. Ayres, 1967; Coelho, 1949; Colson, 1975, Corso, 1953-54; de Josselin de Jong, 1922; Fock, 1967; Karsten, 1915; Métraux, 1963; Roth, 1893; van Gennep, 1909; Voegelin, 1960). Some analysts detect in couvade an assertion of paternity in contexts of matriarchy (Bachofen, 1861; Frazer, 1910; Tylor, 1865, 1889, 1892a, 1892b), among societies characterized by instability of political allegiance in which bride-wealth is emphasized (Paige and Paige, 1981), or under circumstances of psychological uncertainty (Freud, 1942). Others see the essence of the couvade in "parturition envy" (Bettelheim, 1962) or in male claims to reproductive control in "pseudoprocreative" rituals (Hiatt, 1971; Rivière, 1974). That couvade is a form of magical prophylaxis to ensure the well-being of mother and child during birth has also been suggested (Crawley, 1960; Frazer, 1910; Tylor, 1865). Both sex avoidance and food taboos are often emphasized as the focus of the prophylactic measures of couvade (Ayres, 1967). Some emphasize an expression of either empathy (Crawley, 1960) or hostility (Reik, 1931) between husband and wife. Other analysts argue over couvade as either a social dramatization of male parenthood (Young, 1965; Young and Bacdayan, 1965; cf. de Josselin de Jong, 1922; van Gennep, 1909) or a culturally constituted projective outcome of the psychological conflicts of cross-sex identity (Munroe and Munroe, 1971, 1973; Munroe, Munroe, and Nerlove, 1973; Munroe, Munroe, and Whiting, 1965, 1973). In general, nevertheless, it has been the more psychological cast of explanation that has attracted the most attention in clinical attempts to make sense of the couvade symptoms of expectant fathers in the West, where *ritual* couvade is rare (Cavenar and Butts, 1977; Colman and Colman, 1971; Curtis, 1955; Evans, 1951; Freeman, 1951; Ginath, 1974; Gurwitt, 1976; Hogenboom, 1967; Hott, 1976; Jaffe, 1968; Jarvis, 1962; Josselyn, 1956; King, 1968; Munroe and Munroe, 1971; Obrzut, 1976; Polgar, 1963; Rubel and Spielberg, 1966; Spencer, 1949; Trethowan, 1965, 1968, 1972; Trethowan and Conlon, 1965; Wainwright, 1968).

Much anthropological attention has been directed toward ritual couvade as an expression of social structure. Thus, some analysts note that couvade tends to illuminate the distinctiveness of men and women and of the nuclear family as a social unit vis-à-vis the wider society (Colson, 1975; Da Matta, 1971). Others see the relative strength (Briffault, 1931) or fragility (Douglas, 1975) of the marriage bond to be reflected in couvade (cf. Paige and Paige, 1981). Douglas (1975), however, implies that social explanations of couvade are founded on whether the father's ritual is focused primarily on his relationship with the mother (Diaz, 1965) or with the child (Lévi-Strauss, 1962; Métraux, 1963). Yet analytical unity amidst the phenomenal cross-cultural diversity of couvade, whether by construction of multiple typologies (Frazer, 1910; Ploss, 1911; Schmidt, 1954) or putatively universal essential features (Driver, 1969; Munroe, Munroe, and Whiting, 1973), remains elusive. The scope of couvade phenomena may be suggested in Coelho's assertion that, "The couvade is but part of a unified world-view as it regards the interaction of the spiritual realm and the everyday life of man, and of the relations between husband and wife, between father, mother and child" (1949, p. 51). Kroeber, nevertheless, notes that, "The common factor is the name, plus a vague and extremely plastic concept . . . almost as near to a train of related but free associations as to a scientific theory" (1948, p. 543). If the phenomenological, functional, and distributional problems of couvade seem to reflect more the order of family resemblance than of monothetic definition, perhaps analytical advance must be made by approaching such psychocultural phenomena from a particular perspective and by permitting the framework of analysis to provide the significant contours and canons of closure in exploring couvade. The perspective taken here suggests that couvade phenomena may have particular diagnostic, prognostic, and therapeutic functions and, therefore, may present an analytical problem for ethnomedical studies.

This essay explores only a single ethnographical case, but the analytical approach is distinctive. I suggest that Bimin-Kuskusmin couvade ritual may be analyzed as a delicate, adjustable "therapeutic model" that has a variety of diagnostic, prognostic, preventative, curative, and other symbolic functions. Couvade phenomena do not label a specific illness but rather provide a sensitive cultural barometer of *potential* illness in certain social persons involved in the life-crisis of birth. The couvade "model" reveals a cultural construction of birth-related phenomena in terms of which certain individual experiences, stresses, and *consequent* illnesses of particular social people can be predicted, interpreted, and managed. It provides formal recognition of those people, who, by virtue of social identity and individual "case history," are variably vulnerable to stress and illness during pregnancy, birth, and thereafter. It permits preventative and therapeutic measures to be taken in alleviating stress and preventing or curing illness in afflicted people. Curers may expand and contract the number, intensity, and duration of many behavioral restrictions for the focal father and mother, and other couvade ritual participants may impose on the father, mother, or themselves further variations in the kinds and degrees of ritual taboos. As vulnerability to stress and illness of the father, mother, and infant is seen to increase or decrease with the normal process of pregnancy, birth, and postpartum events (and under special circumstances), the sphere of kin participating in couvade also expands and contracts. This cognatic sphere of kin, who act as both participants and decision makers in Bimin-Kuskusmin ritual couvade, may be analyzed in terms of what Janzen (1978) calls "therapy managing groups." Of particular importance, however, the Bimin-Kuskusmin case provides an instance in which couvade ritual and couvade symptoms are explicitly articulated. This articulation has significant implications for an understanding of the adverse reactions of Bimin-Kuskusmin, who recognize birth-related illnesses in males, to the gynecological-obstetrical services of local Western clinics, which ignore or reject their view and diagnose such male "symptoms" as manifestations of diverse diseases.[5] Although this mode of analysis of couvade phenomena may prove to be useful elsewhere in Melanesia (cf. Blackwood, 1935; Glick, 1963; Hayano, 1974; Hogbin, 1943, 1970; Malinowski, 1927; Mead, 1970; Meigs, 1976; Pospisil, 1978; Powdermaker, 1971) and perhaps more generally, this investigation is embedded in the ethnography of the Bimin-Kuskusmin, whom I shall briefly introduce.

THE BIMIN-KUSKUSMIN: AN ETHNOGRAPHIC INTRODUCTION

About one thousand Bimin-Kuskusmin occupy a rugged, ecologically diverse, mountainous area in the southeastern West Sepik Province of Papua New Guinea (Figure I). Speaking a Mountain-Ok language, they note with pride their uniqueness and historical primacy in the region. Networks of trade, intermarriage, alliance, warfare, and ritual relations, however, bring them into contact with other ethnic groups of the area. They have known of the European at least since the Kaiserin-Augusta-Fluss Expedition (1912-1914) penetrated the Telefomin region to the west. First direct contact with Europeans, however, was experienced by only a few people in 1957. During the next several years, they endured a number of devastating influenza epidemics that killed many and terrified all. Influenza became the first instance of an emerging category of "European illnesses," which later came to include mumps, measles, and whooping cough. In the early 1960s, government and mission clinics were established among the Oksapmin people to the north, and occasional medical patrols began to probe the periphery of Bimin-Kuskusmin territory. On

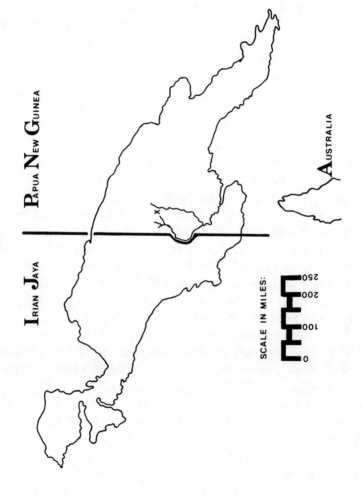

FIGURE I
The Island of New Guinea
X: The Bimin-Kuskusmin

IRIAN JAVA

PAPUA NEW GUINEA

AUSTRALIA

SCALE IN MILES:

0 100 200 250

the eve of fieldwork in 1971, nevertheless, familiarity with government and mission custom remained slight and laden with suspicion and fear.

Much of the daily round is spent in sexually segregated subsistence activities. Men cultivate taro and nut pandanus, tend banana and other semicultivated crops, and hunt or trap a variety of forest game. Women cultivate sweet potato and other domestic food plants and gather wild faunae and florae in forest and stream. A few feral dogs, cassowary chicks, and pigs are captured by men but are tended by women. Most foods are categorized as "male" (*kunum* or *imok*) or "female" (*waneng* or *yangus*), and such classification has significance in an elaborate system of food taboos and *materia medica*. The elaboration of gender ideology informs much of Bimin-Kuskusmin social life (Poole, 1981a, 1981b, 1981c).

Bimin-Kuskusmin social structure is conceived in an agnatic idiom with overt recognition of important cognatic, uterine, and affinal links (Poole, 1976b). Lineages and cognatic kindreds are traced through shared "agnatic blood" (*kunum khaim*). Clans, ritual moieties, and initiation age-groups are reckoned in terms of shared *finiik* spirit.[6] Such cultural categories are articulated in complex ways with a range of social groups and transactions and are important in divination, curing, midwifery, and other realms of ritual. Whereas male and female healers are identified with particular clans, a more informal "therapy managing group" (Janzen, 1978) is generally drawn from the patrilineage and cognatic kindred of the afflicted person. Although the partially overlapping kindreds of father, mother, and child are centrally involved in couvade performances,[7] primary ritual control in couvade is vested in a female ritual elder or curer-diviner-midwife of the father's clan (Poole, 1981c), with which the child's primary jural identity is associated. Such postmenopausal women control the formal management of both male couvade phenomena and midwifery at a mother's childbearing.

It is important to note that these ritual "midwives" (*waneng kusem ser*) are highly androgynous in character, as are all Bimin-Kuskusmin at various points of the life-cycle and under varying circumstances (Poole, 1981c). Thus, the ritual midwives are uniquely able to deal with the juxtapositions and combinations of "male" and "female" phenomena that are associated with conception, pregnancy, birth, couvade performances, and couvade illnesses. The traditional Bimin-Kuskusmin understanding of conception,

pregnancy, birth, and related couvade phenomena involves a reckoning of complex and shifting balances of *both* male *and* female
elements. The Bimin-Kuskusmin model of procreation is based on
reckoning the flow of "male" and "female" substances *to* and
through persons. Various aspects of "male" and "female" substances
forge particular dimensions of anatomy, spirit, social identity, and
personality. It is this flow of differentiated substances that links a
man and a woman in different ways to their unborn child and in
similar ways to their different, exogamous kindreds, which partially
overlap with the kindred of the child. It is by virtue of their
substantial links to the fragile unborn or newborn infant that both
parents are considered to be vulnerable to various illnesses before,
during, and after birth events. Furthermore, the essential "therapy
managing group" (Janzen, 1978) for both parents and child at such
times of birth-related vulnerability is ideally formed by at least one
member of each of the following lineage categories: both mother's
and father's own lineages and the lineages of their respective
mothers, fathers' mothers, and mothers' mothers, which together
constitute the cognatic kindred of the child. Finally, much of the
idiom of couvade ritual observances and of the delicate adjustments
in couvade "therapy" is interwoven with notions of procreative
substances and processes.

The idea of *balance* of substance is crucial, for almost all ailments are recognized as an imbalance of corporeal and noncorporeal
dimensions of the person — dimensions that are laid down in procreation and transformed, negated, or supplemented throughout the life
cycle by means of "natural" maturation, the ingestion of "male"
and "female" foods, and ritual intervention in "natural" processes
of development. Illness represents a balance that is diagnostic of a
particular affliction, but an imbalance vis-à-vis the sick person's
proper sociocultural identity by virtue of age, sex, marital status,
parenthood, and ritual rank. There is no term for "illness" per se in
the Bimin-Kuskusmin language, but the classification of particular
maladies is permeated by a notion of "external" (*bangep*) and
"internal" (*mutuuk*) worries or troubles (*sakhiik*), which are believed
to cause substantial or spiritual imbalances in the person. Although
both aspects of anxiety tend to be interwoven in any particular
instance, external troubles generally refer to malaise or misfortune
in economic, political, religious, and other social matters that have
untoward consequences for the person. Internal worries, however,

refer to the disruption of psychobiological and spiritual balances within the person, often as either (or both) consequence or (and) cause of external troubles. Diagnostic divination seeks to articulate the "external" and the "internal" features of anxiety through attention to a person's "case history," diagnosis of special vulnerabilities or extant illnesses, and prognostic therapeutic intervention vis-à-vis both the person and the relevant social milieu. Divination proceeds, however, from an assessment of imbalances in the person as a bodily and spiritual entity made up of components, processes, and capacities that are first forged in procreation, transformed both "naturally" and ritually over the course of the life cycle, and then occasionally altered through the stress of particular life crises. It is in this general context of traditional belief that couvade ritual must be perceived.

PREGNANCY AND PRENATAL COUVADE

Since the menstrual cycles of Bimin-Kuskusmin women may· be notably irregular on occasion,[8] a prolonged cessation of menstruation is not always considered to be indicative of pregnancy. Despite possible suspicions, the husband continues his routine behavior until his wife has privately consulted a midwife of his clan. If the divination is positive, the wife publicly announces her pregnancy early in the second trimester. Then, the midwife declares that the expectant father is subject to the formal restrictions of the "sacred womb rite" (*men am ben aiyem*). The expectant father must now refrain from many routine activities. While continuing to reside in a men's house and to engage in male subsistence activities, he must avoid male ritual events and all women (except those who are pregnant) and all children. Indeed, he is considered to be highly polluting to all people except initiated men, pregnant women, and female ritual elders. In order to provide emotional support for his wife and to ensure the proper growth of the unborn child, however, he must caress his wife's abdomen daily, and they must have sexual intercourse with increasing frequency during the second and early third trimesters. His semen will enhance the strength and general prenatal development of the child and will increase the probability of a son. Yet, frequent intercourse is extremely debilitating.[9] To ensure the strength of his body and semen, he is subject to numerous divinations and treatments of any illnesses or wounds that exude pus, which is believed to be a manifestation of semen. He must conserve his energy through increasing inactivity. He must shun all places where dangerous forest spirits or witches abound, for they will weaken his male substance. He must avoid contact with women and children under most circumstances, for their pollution is now especially dangerous to him. He should avoid "female" foods but consume large amounts of "male" foods that contain *finiik* spirit, which is the active force in semen.

For expectant fathers, especially those who are themselves first-born sons and who have no children or only daughters, the kinds and amounts of "male" foods (especially pork, taro, and nut pandanus) that are eaten during the prenatal couvade increase considerably. In such cases, and in cases of men whose wives have experienced childbirth difficulties or have produced sons with genital abnormalities, the men's lineage brothers also increase their consumption of "male" foods. Strict taboos are placed, however, on those "male" foods that are believed to interfere with the well-being of mother and child or to impede proper prenatal development and birth. Thus, for a variety of supernatural reasons, men must avoid all snakes, all florae and faunae that are associated with water and are "cold" (*giriir*), all burrowing animals except the sacred spiny anteater, certain birds with long or sharp beaks, and certain mammals that escape from traps by severing an appendage or cling tenaciously to their prey.

If any of these couvade food taboos are broken, cognatic kin of the expectant father, who are not also of the child's kindred, deliberately eat the forbidden food to deflect the supernatural consequences away from the father, mother, and child. In turn, cognatic kin of the expectant father, who are also of the child's kindred, conduct sacrifices to remedy the situation, and they too begin to observe some of the father's food restrictions. Food taboos among these two sets of cognatic kin, however, will vary according to the circumstances of the father's breach of taboo and will always be less in number, intensity, and duration than those of the father. The most severe restrictions will fall on men of the father's own lineage, with less on his mother's and father's mother's lineages and least on his mother's mother's lineage. As food taboos decrease with the outward radiation of the father's ego-centered kindred, so does the number and the kind and degree of involvement of the participants. The father's patrilineal and matrilateral lineages are usually well represented, but there is sometimes no more than a single participant from each of the other lineages (father's mother's and mother's mother's). If any of the latter are not represented, however, the father's well-being, and indirectly that of mother and child, are more at risk. Thus, more close cognatic kin of the father must assume limited couvade restrictions. They are said to form a "shield" (*askom*) between the increasingly vulnerable father (and, through him, mother and child) and the potentially dangerous, nonpartici- pating, distant cognatic kin.[10]

Although, in contrast, the lineage representatives are female, "male" foods are forbidden, and "female" foods are prescribed, the same kinds of graded observances pertain to that sector of the mother's kindred that overlaps with the kindred of her unborn child. Siblings of the unborn infant, however, are not subject to couvade restrictions at this time, although both the youngest (being "closest to the womb") and eldest (being representative of the sibling set) may take on a few minor food taboos voluntarily. The mother's co-wives often take on themselves a few token restrictions. They are believed to be jealous of and hostile toward the pregnant mother, for her pregnancy denies them sexual attention from the father. Should a son be born, he will compete with their sons for the father's favor. Should a daughter be born, she will compete with their daugh- ters for the father's support in arranging the best marriages, and the bridewealth gained in her marriage will be devoted to her actual brothers' marriages. Thus, the minimal participation of co-wives in couvade is expected to signal only a grudging support; and if there should be misfortune during the forthcoming birth, they are less vulnerable to accusations of witchcraft on account of their participation.

Prenatal development of the "fetus" (*aur kumun*) is monitored in several ways. First, the father's clan midwife divines its condition through palpation of the mother's abdomen, examination of her own reflection in the mother's eyes, and scrutiny of the contents of the intestines of certain marsupials. Second, male members of the patrilineal and matrilateral lineages of *both* mother *and* father collectively divine fetal development through examination of the father's reflection in a pool of pig's blood to determine the strength of certain "male" aspects of the constitution of the unborn child. Third, the father, who has been touching his wife's abdomen regu- larly, makes his own assessment of prenatal development on the basis of the size, shape, elevation, and relative softness of the swollen abdomen. Fourth, a lineage brother of the father who is participating in prenatal couvade restrictions divines the contents of the intestines of both a tree-nesting and a ground-nesting bird to determine the position of the child in the womb at the time of birth relative to its present position. When these four modes of divination are in agreement on the advanced stage of growth of the fetus (in about the middle of the last trimester), sexual intercourse must cease abruptly. Its continuance would threaten the "female" parts of the anatomy and prized external appearance of the child and might also damage certain "female" parts of the mother's anatomy that are central to the process of giving birth.

At this critical point, the father's vulnerability to illness is thought to increase dramatically and his couvade restrictions begin to change. Polluted by "female" foods, "female" bodily substances, and intimate involvement with childbearing, he must now withdraw from *all* male contact and activity and must sleep deep in the forest or in a remote garden hut. The "female name" (*waneng win*) of his childhood before male initiation must now be used exclusively. His upper torso is covered with protective white pigment mixed with sow fat to guard against illness.[11] Both the father and his *entire* kindred now abandon strong "male" foods and consume only soft and weak "female" foods. In contrast, the mother and that sphere of her kindred that overlaps the kindred of the child forsake "female" foods and begin to eat only increasingly strong "male" foods.

In prenatal couvade, there is a complementarity between father and mother vis-à-vis the unborn infant. Through procreative process, both parents have transmitted separate, but complementary substances to the child, have forged male and female aspects of the corporeal and noncorporeal identity of the child, and have linked the child to patrilateral and matrilateral sets of cognatic kin who will form its kindred. Yet, the balance is asymmetrical, for the father is responsible for establishing the stronger "male" anatomy, *finiik* spirit, "agnatic blood," and bonds of patrilineal descent and patrifiliation of the child. In contrast, during the pregnancy, the father becomes weaker and more vulnerable to illnesses than the mother. At first, the mother and her close cognatic kin (female) emphasize their femaleness through numerous couvade restrictions but largely continue their routine activities. The father and his close cognatic kin (male) emphasize their maleness, and the father withdraws from routine activities to observe increasingly restrictive couvade taboos and to strut his enhanced sexuality and potency. While the mother remains more passive in reinforcing the "female" anatomy of the child through "female" foods, the father more aggressively strengthens its "male" anatomy and attempts to create a son through augmented semen and sexual prowess. The father's semen and diet of "male" foods are said to strengthen the child's "heart" (*iboorop*) and "bone" (*kuun*), which are symbols of the "male" anatomy. The mother's fertile fluids, menstrual blood, and diet of "female" foods are believed to strengthen the child's "fat" (*tukhuur*) and "skin" (*kaar*), which are symbols of the "female anatomy.

Then, at the cessation of sexual intercourse, the emphasis shifts. Now the depleted father, having expended his potency, increasingly retires into a more passive female and in some ways childlike role, as do his cognatic kin. As his cognatic kin become somewhat freer to engage in routine activities, however, it is now his entire kindred that is represented in couvade observances. That is, the intensity of involvement declines as the extent of social participation expands, which is a common mechanism for achieving various aspects of ritual balance in Bimin-Kuskusmin couvade. At this stage, however, the father's vulnerability to illness has notably increased. In marked contrast, the mother (and the cognatic kin whom she shares with her unborn infant), now preparing for the rigors of childbearing, increasingly emphasizes her "male" strength and endurance through strenuous activity and adherence to food taboos that emphasize the consumption of "male" foods and the invigoration of her "male" anatomy.

SECLUSION, LABOR, BIRTH, AND COUVADE

When his wife's first labor contractions are announced by the midwife of his clan, the father goes into strict seclusion in the forest of his clan's land. His seclusion coincides with that of his wife in a "birth hut" (*singiiam*). Although his lineage brothers continue to supply his "female" foods, only the androgynous midwife may now approach him without subsequently undergoing elaborate rites of purification. Until the birth, the father continues to cover his upper body with white pigment and to observe his "female" food taboos. He is now subject, however, to further couvade restrictions.

He must shed his phallocrypt and remain naked as a sign of his lack of sexuality and potency and his childlike status (cf. Lévi-Strauss, 1962). He is denied fire in order not to draw heat away from mother and child at this critical time and to emphasize the feral aspects of his condition. He may neither uproot nor plant anything in order to avoid premature or breech delivery and to emphasize his feral dependance on wild foods (such as berries and nuts) that can be gathered above ground. New prescriptions of particular "female" foods are believed to ensure a quick and easy birth, a fine external appearance for the child as reflected in fatness and a glistening skin, and some protection from menstrual pollution for both mother and child.

The consumption of these new "female" foods, however, is said to increase markedly the father's vulnerability to virulent "black blood" (*khaim mighiir*) illnesses, which are associated with the menstrual pollution that he draws away from mother and child and toward himself. In fact, perhaps due to some combination of radically altered diet, inactivity, exposure, and other forms of physical and psychological stress, most fathers almost invariably experience some discernible ailment by this stage of *couvade*. On the basis of the father's "case history" (especially with respect to prior experience of birth events) and meticulous divination of emerging symptoms, certain preventative and therapeutic measures are taken. Generally, the father's close cognatic kin impose additional food prescriptions on the father, themselves, or both. The white flesh of certain nuts, fruits, or tubers is usually included, for the color white in a moist medium, whether in a food or represented by white pigment and sow fat, is believed to possess strong curative powers. In cases of serious illness, such kin may make sacrifices to the father's clan ancestors and his clan midwife may increase the father's food prescriptions or take on herself his full complement of food taboos. On occasion, she may add a particular food that has special curative significance in the context of the father's case history, his clan, his particular illness, her reputation, or oddities present in the prior constellation of his food prescriptions. Divinations and dietary adjustments may be numerous and intricate and may involve strategic expansions and contractions of the "therapy managing group" of cognatic kin, who ritually envelop the vulnerable father, in terms of both the extent and the kind of participation in couvade observances.

When the father is formally told of his wife's seclusion, he refrains from any water or food, except cucumber and sugarcane, until the birth. During this time, he eats morsels of psychogenic fungi to produce visions, rubs himself with stinging-nettle leaves to cause painful welts to form, and offers prayers to his clan ancestors for a healthy son. He tries to focus his dreams on male phenomena, such as ritual implements, acts of warfare, or boar hunting, to exert some final influence over the determination of sex. He scans the forest for omens of a normal delivery and a male child. His entire kindred continues to eat "female" foods. Initiated siblings of the unborn child, both male and female, now also assume these couvade restrictions, but in a graded manner according to gender and full or half siblingship. The father's lineage and clan sisters now also participate, and for the first time, with the sole exception of the clan midwife, the father's female kin enter couvade restrictions. In contrast, the mother's cognatic kin, both male and female, continue to eat "male" foods, but the male participants are both restricted in number and newly introduced into the sphere of couvade observances. The most important male participants, nevertheless, are her close patrilineal kinsmen. Her father must now gorge himself on strong "male" foods to ensure the strength of her "fertile fluids" (*mem gom*), for which he is procreatively responsible. If there are birth difficulties, the midwife of her husband's clan may prescribe further specialized "male" foods for her father, especially the bone marrow from wild boars or the heart of a cassowary. If her father vomits from appropriately gorging himself, however, the birth will be easier. In addition to her lineage brothers, who consume "male" foods and ritually control her hemorrhaging during childbearing, the mother's father is her only formally participating kinsman. Her male cognatic kin usually also consume some "male" foods, but they do so informally on the basis of amity and moral concern and not of jural or ritual obligation.

During couvade ritual at birth, the mother and the father are joined in the pangs of fasting and in the pain of rubbing themselves with harsh stinging-nettle leaves. As the father struggles to control his *finiik* spirit in dreams and visions and his clan ancestors' attention to the event through prayers and as the mother struggles to control the physical process of childbearing, there is an increasing ritual focus on the child. The couvade observances of cognatic kin of the mother and child, of the father and child, and of the father now differ markedly from those of the fasting, suffering mother and father, who must be protectively "enveloped" (*emkhreykhai'ookhasey*) by these three sets of cognatic kin. Thus, the mother's father and brothers and the father's mother and sisters now expand the "therapy managing group." The child, however, also becomes of central concern. This new focus is particularly marked by the formal couvade participation of the child's initiated male and female siblings and by the beginning of several new couvade observances of the father. First, he applies white pigment to his abdomen, which is said to have become swollen and painful, in the manner of his similarly adorned wife in order to protect the child against illness, witchcraft, wandering spirits, and ancestral spirits of unavenged warriors. Second, he cuts his navel and smears the blood on his penis to facilitate the child's "detachment" (*akaraak'nam*) from the mother's womb and "attachment" (*adetera'fefebaanam*) to his agnatic kin and ancestral clan land. Third, he assumes a squatting position and violently contracts his viscera, often defecating or urinating in his efforts, to facilitate an easy delivery for the mother and child. Upon the formal announcement of the birth, however, the new father's couvade observances change abruptly.

POSTNATAL COUVADE

If the birth results in a stillborn child or a deformed infant that must be strangled or twins, one of which must be killed, the father must continue the severe couvade restrictions that he has assumed during the process of labor and birth. Such continuation of couvade restrictions is also the case if his wife dies in childbirth, which presumes the death or strangulation of the newborn. In these cases, he will be slowly reintroduced to powerful "male" foods and will be carefully monitored through divination by both male and female clan curers. Much attention will be directed toward the prevention of suicide, to which he is believed to be especially prone under the unfortunate circumstances.

With the birth of a normal son or daughter, however, the father abandons his isolated retreat in the forest and slowly begins to reenter the social community. His food restrictions immediately shift to the prenatal emphasis on "male" foods and the denial of "female" foods. These observances may continue for a period of time, for he is thought to be still highly vulnerable to illness and depression. It is said, nevertheless, that his masculine strength, founded on a replenishment of "male" substance through his altered diet, will soon return. As he now secretly approaches the polluted birth hut of his wife and child, the midwife presents his newborn infant to him. Alone, he takes the child to a nearby stream of ancestral significance to his clan to wash it and then to place some of the white pigment that clings to his body on its face in order to protect the infant and to enhance its beauty. He annoints the infant with sow fat to ward off the cold and wandering spirits or witches. He may bestow on his child a secret name that is drawn from some natural phenomena near the stream and that only he will know and share with the clan ancestors until the child ceremonially receives a formal "female name" at the appearance of deciduous teeth. Returning the infant to the midwife, he washes, purifies himself with stinging-nettle leaves and boar fat, and once again puts on a phallocrypt, which is now decorated with symbols of the gender of the child. He now reenters his men's house, but he is forbidden to hunt, to enter his taro garden, or to engage in male ritual activities until his strength has returned and most of his couvade restrictions have been lifted. He may not see his secluded wife and child for several days. As the child begins to nurse, the mother will gradually begin to shed her couvade food taboos and resume a regular adult woman's diet. For several years until full weaning has occurred, however, she will continue to eat certain prescribed "male" foods and will observe a postpartum sex taboo in order to enhance the strength of her breast milk.

At this time, all initiated males of the child's entire kindred are obliged to eat some "male" foods to ensure the strength, well-being, and proper development of the infant. As the food taboos of the mother and father gradually decrease, those of the child's cognatic kin increase until the bestowal of a "female name" on the child. All of the child's kindred who are subject to any couvade restrictions, except the mother and father, are forbidden to touch the infant, who is precariously fragile. When the mother and child emerge from seclusion, the first to be released from these restrictions are the initiated siblings and both sets of grandparents. They are the first people except the parents to hold and to play with the child, with whom they will continue a close, affectionate relationship for life. Soon thereafter, most couvade restrictions are quickly removed from all cognatic kin unless the infant should fall ill, but those restrictions in force on the father and his male lineage agnates endure.

The new father is still highly contaminating to himself and to others, and both kith and kin (male and female) must avoid direct contact with him or his bodily and food leavings. Only the clan midwife who attended the birth and other female ritual elders of his clan are immune to his pollution. Despite his now constant consumption of "male" foods and his endurance of a succession of rites of purification, his strength and masculine purity are said to be slow to return. Thus, until divination by the midwife indicates that he has passed a critical threshold of recovery from his ordeal, he is forbidden to have sexual intercourse to ensure that he does not endanger the progress of his recovery. Indeed, the postpartum sex taboo would forbid sexual access to the wife who gave birth to his newest child, and unless he is married polygynously, he would not have legitimate sexual access to any other woman. He would also be forbidden to masturbate, however, for such acts would deplete his strength in the same manner as sexual intercourse. Similarly, he must take special care to avoid injuring himself and must carefully tend all wounds, for the loss of pus is considered to be equivalent to the loss of semen, of which pus is a manifestation.

In his present condition, the father is still considered to be fragile, weak, and prone to illness, as is his newborn child. He is said to be filled with "internal worry" (*sakhiik mutuuk*) over the health of the infant despite the success of childbirth.[12] Consequently, he is thought to be quick to anger and easily depressed. Other couvade symptoms of the father in Bimin-Kuskusmin reckoning include lassitude, weakness, shortness of breath, pronounced increase in appetite or anorexia, leg or abdominal cramps, abdominal distention and pain, nausea, bloody diarrhea, headaches, and fever. For those fathers who have lost a wife or child, either during the present birth event or even in prior experience, however, couvade symptoms are said to be most severe and often to culminate in suicidal depression, especially if the loss has occurred during the present birth event. In such cases, the full force and scope of prenatal couvade restrictions are reimposed on the man, and with the stillbirth or strangulation of the infant of the present birth event, the most severe restrictions of couvade during the process of birth may also be reimposed. His cognatic kin, who also resume their couvade observances under these circumstances, never permit him to be left alone. In one of the 37 cases of couvade on which I have extensive data, a man who had experienced the deaths of two wives in childbirth (one dying in the

TABLE I
Aspects of 37 Case Histories of Couvade Symptoms among Bimin-Kuskusmin Men

Characteristics of "Fathers"	Cases																		
	1	2	3	4	5	6	7	8	9	10	11	12	13	14	15	16	17	18	19
Prior or Other Wives (not including the wife who is involved in the present birth event)																			
Married Previously or Polygynously to Other Wives – No. of Prior or Other Wives	0	1	0	3	1	0	0	0	4	0	0	1	0	0	0	0	0	0	2
No. of Pregnancies by Prior/Other Wives[a]	0	3	0	7	4	0	0	0	0	0	0	2	0	0	0	0	0	0	6
No. of Live Births by Prior/Other Wives[b]	0	2	0	5	2	0	0	0	0	0	0	2	0	0	0	0	0	0	5
No. of Stillbirths by Prior/Other Wives[c]	0	1	0	1	1	0	0	0	0	0	0	0	0	0	0	0	0	0	0
No. of Twin Births by Prior/Other Wives[d]	0	0	0	0	0	0	0	0	0	0	0	0	0	0	0	0	0	0	0
No. of Abnormal Births by Prior/Other Wives (refers to the abnormal characteristics of the child)	0	0	0	1	1	0	0	0	0	0	0	1	0	0	0	0	0	0	1
No. of Childbirth Complications (for prior/other wives)	0	1	0	1	2	0	0	0	0	0	0	1	0	0	0	0	0	0	3
No. of Childbirth Fatalities (of prior/other wives)	0	0	0	1	1	0	0	0	0	0	0	0	0	0	0	0	0	0	1
No. of Surviving Children by Prior/Other Wives[e]	M0/F1	M0/F1	0	M0/F1	M1/F0	0	0	0	0	0	0	M1/F0	0	0	0	0	0	0	M3/F1
Present Wife (the wife who is involved in the present birth event)																			
No. of Pregnancies by Present Wife – Prior Pregnancies	1	2	0	0	2	1	0	0	0	1	2	0	3	0	0	0	0	1	0
No. of Live Births by Present Wife	1	2	0	0	1	1	0	0	0	1	2	0	2	0	0	0	0	1	0
No. of Stillbirths by Present Wife	0	0	0	0	1	0	0	0	0	0	0	0	1	0	0	0	0	0	0
No. of Twin Births by Present Wife	0	0	0	0	0	0	0	0	0	0	0	0	0	0	0	0	0	0	0
No. of Abnormal Births by Present Wife (refers to the abnormal characteristics of the child)	0	0	0	0	1	0	0	0	0	0	0	0	0	0	0	0	0	0	0
No. of Childbirth Complications (for present wife)	1	0	0	0	1	0	0	0	0	1	1	0	1	0	0	0	0	0	0

72

Childbirth Fatality of Present Wife	0	0	0	0	0	0	0	0	0	0	0	X
No. of Surviving Children by Present Wife	M1 F0	M1 F1	M1 F0	M0 F1	M1 F0	M0 F1	M1 F1	M0 F1	M1 F0	M1 F1	M0 F1	M0 F1
Prior Experience of "Couvade Symptoms" by the Father[f]	(3)	(1) 0	(1)	(1) (2) 0	(3)	(1) 0	(3) (2) (1) 0	(1)	(2) (1) 0	(3)	0 0	(1)

(continued)

TABLE I, continued

Characteristics of "Fathers"	Cases																	
	20	21	22	23	24	25	26	27	28	29	30	31	32	33	34	35	36	37
Prior or Other Wives (not including the wife who is involved in the present birth event)																		
Married Previously or Polygynously to Other Wives – No. of Prior or Other Wives	0	0	1	1	0	0	1	1	2	0	1	0	0	0	0	0	1	0
No. of Pregnancies by Prior/Other Wives[a]	0	0	4	3	0	0	0	5	6	0	3	0	0	0	0	0	1	0
No. of Live Births by Prior/Other Wives[b]	0	0	3	3	0	0	0	4	5	0	3	0	0	0	0	0	1	0
No. of Stillbirths by Prior/Other Wives[c]	0	0	1	0	0	0	0	1	0	0	0	0	0	0	0	0	0	0
No. of Twin Births by Prior/Other Wives[d]	0	0	0	0	0	0	0	1	0	0	0	0	0	0	0	0	0	0
No. of Abnormal Births by Prior/Other Wives (refers to the abnormal characteristics of the child)	0	0	0	1	0	0	0	1	0	0	0	0	0	0	0	0	0	0
No. of Childbirth Complications (for prior/other wives)	0	0	2	1	0	0	0	2	0	0	0	0	0	0	0	0	0	0
No. of Childbirth Fatalities (of prior/other wives)	0	0	0	0	0	0	0	1	1	0	0	0	0	0	0	0	0	0
No. of Surviving Children by Prior/Other Wives[e]	0	0	M1 F1	M0 F2	0	0	0	M1 F1	M1 F2	0	M3 F0	0	0	0	0	0	M1 F0	0
Present Wife (the wife who is involved in the present birth event)																		
No. of Pregnancies by Present Wife – Prior Pregnancies	2	3	1	0	0	0	1	4	1	2	0	0	3	2	0	1	0	0
No. of Live Births by Present Wife	1	3	1	0	0	0	0	3	1	1	0	0	3	2	0	1	0	0
No. of Stillbirths by Present Wife	0	0	0	0	0	0	1	0	0	1	0	0	0	0	0	0	0	0
No. of Twin Births by Present Wife	0	0	0	0	0	0	0	0	0	0	0	0	0	0	0	0	0	0
No. of Abnormal Births by Present Wife (refers to the abnormal characteristics of the child)	1	0	0	0	0	0	1	1	0	0	0	0	1	1	0	0	0	0
No. of Childbirth Complications (for present wife)	1	0	0	0	0	0	0	1	0	1	0	0	1	1	0	0	0	0

74

Childbirth Fatality of Present Wife	0	0	0	0	X	0	0	0	0	X	0	0	0	0	X	0	0
No. of Surviving Children by Present Wife	M0 F1	M2 F1	M1 F0			M2 F0	M0 F1	M0 F1			M1 F2	M0 F1	M1 F0				
Prior Experience of *"Couvade Symptoms"* by the Father[f]	(2)	0	0	(1)	(3)	0	(1)	(1)	(1)	0	(2)	(3)	(1)	(3)	0	(3)	(2)

Notes:

[a]This number is probably a minimum. Pregnancies not resulting in live births are not usually recorded in genealogies or life histories and are quite difficult to reconstruct even if they are quite recent. Such information is drawn, therefore, from delicate, private interviews.

[b]The reckoning of live births assumes survival of the infant until the appearance of deciduous teeth (at 20 to 24 months for complete temporary dentition) and the ceremonial bestowal of "female names." Unnamed infants who perish are often classified with the stillborn by Bimin-Kuskusmin and may be distinguished only through delicate, private interviews.

[c]Stillbirths (often including early infant deaths) are very difficult to elicit, and this number is probably a minimum. The same is true of those abnormal newborn infants who are killed. Blame, guilt, shame, and supernatural sanctions are usually associated with all such ill-fated births.

[d]Due perhaps to the special supernatural implications of their appearance, twin births appear to be elicited more readily.

[e]F = female; M = male.

[f]The relative severity of couvade "symptoms" is classified in accordance with Bimin-Kuskusmin reckoning as "serious" [(3)], "less serious" [(2)], "least serious" [(3)], and "no symptoms acknowledged" [(0)].

birth under investigation) committed suicide before leaving his seclusion in the forest (see Table I: case 19). Thus, the alteration, removal, and reimposition of the father's couvade observances is delicately regulated by divinatory and other social perceptions — within his lineage, clan (as represented by the midwife), and kindred — of the linked vulnerabilities of father, mother, and child. Divinatory diagnosis of the father's condition by the clan midwife, the "therapy managing group" of his kindred, and the more private deliberations of his lineage agnates, therefore, is focused on five primary factors: (1) the postpartum health of the infant; (2) the postpartum health of his wife; (3) the postpartum increase in his masculine strength and purity; (4) his "case history," especially in regard to his prior experiences of childbirth; and (5) his particular social identity.

If all is well, however, the father's couvade restrictions are lifted several days after the birth of a daughter; but they are usually observed for a longer period if the newborn daughter is a firstborn child or a firstborn or only daughter. In the case of a son, the father's restrictions continue for a full lunar cycle; and if the son is a firstborn son, they persist for almost two lunar cycles. In the case of a firstborn son who is also a firstborn child, however, at least some couvade restrictions remain in force for the father until the child has received a "female name" and the father has adopted a teknonym that incorporates that name. As Fortes (1974, 1978) notes, the position of the firstborn is special. A firstborn child, whether male or female, is welcomed by Bimin-Kuskusmin, for its appearance alters the moral and jural status of both parents-to-be. In some ways, however, parenthood is not complete without both a daugher and a son. Yet, it is the firstborn son who is the firstborn par excellence and the symbolic assurance of his father's potential status as a lineage founder and his eventual enshrinement as an ancestor. Thus, the father who does not have a son and, secondarily, a daughter, and especially the man who is childless, is thought to be particularly prone to unusual stress in the context of his wife's childbearing. Such a father who is himself a firstborn son is perhaps under the greatest stress, for he is said to have jural advantage in succession to rank in the Bimin-Kuskusmin ritual commissions, positions that are predicated on being the father of a son. So, on occasion, such men may even observe limited couvade restrictions until their firstborn sons are first initiated (ideally at 9 to 12 years of age).

The final lifting of couvade ritual taboos from the new father involves both special divinations and formal presentations to kin who have participated in couvade. When it is agreed that the father "appears" to be well and strong again, his clan midwife and cognatic "therapy managing group" jointly conduct an elaborate divination of his reflection in a pool of boar's blood, which is supplied by his male lineage agnates. Significant patterns of seeds, nuts, and pieces of polished wood floating across or sinking beneath parts of his reflection are cosidered to be indicative of the anatomical locus of the affliction. If divination reveals inauspicious signs of dangerous maladies in vital "male" or "female" organs, particular couvade observances, focused on "male" or "female" foods having particular affinity for the afflicted organ(s), may be continued, reimposed, or added anew. In such cases, further divinations will occur to monitor the course of the ailment and to provide the basis for continuances or readjustments of couvade restrictions. Finally, if such diagnosis suggests that all is well, all restrictions are lifted from the father upon completion of certain formal couvade presentations to kin.

In reciprocity for their couvade participation, the father must make specific presentations not only to his wife, lineage agnates, and clan midwife but also to the child's mother's sister, mother's brother, mother's mother, and mother's father. Presentations to other members of his own, his wife's, and his child's cognatic kin are made later and more informally. These presentations consist of particular, symbolically significant valuables, foods, and ritual objects. They not only acknowledge the gender and health of the child, the fecundity of the mother, and those responsible for both but also position the child with respect to a supportive network of close cognatic kin. These prestations and the lifting of couvade restrictions from the father shift attention to the child as an increasingly social person and member of a widening community of kin. Thereafter, the developing personhood (Fortes, 1973) of the child will be marked by a succession of childhood rites of passage that lead into the elaborate initiation rituals of adulthood and that effect a child's confrontation of the cultural constellation of the self (Harris, 1978). Should the child become ill, however, the father may reinstitute certain couvade observances on his own initiative and in accordance with the severity of the ailment. Once children are formally initiated, however, different therapeutic measures appropriate to their more or less adult status will be used. Only when the child itself becomes a parent, will the father once again enter into couvade ritual in order to protect it from harm.

VULNERABILITY AND COUVADE SYMPTOMS

In general, the "sacred womb rite" is formal and socially prescribed. Proper observance of couvade ritual prescriptions is both a jural and a moral obligation of kinship, and breach of couvade taboos is a serious and negatively sanctioned matter of deep "shame" (*fiitom*), demanding atonement and compensation to the injured persons. The participation of the couvade "therapy managing group" is essential, for some fathers are seen as being especially vulnerable to birth-related stress. Such men exhibit recognized constellations of significant symptoms that are immediately obvious or discernible through specialized divination. The appropriate therapeutic adjustments in the prescriptions and proscriptions of the "sacred womb rite" are based on complaints or divinations of these patterns of symptoms. Bimin-Kuskusmin recognize three key grades of such couvade symptoms: (1) serious, including shortness of breath, anorexia, bloody diarrhea, and high fever; (2) less serious, including leg or abdominal cramps, abdominal distention and pain, and nausea; and (3) least serious, including lassitude, weakness, some increase in appetite, and headaches. I have collected extensive data on 37 cases of such couvade symptoms (Table I) through which to explore some aspects of this more variable recognition of male vulnerability during birth events.

In the focal 37 cases, 12 men exhibited serious; 5, less serious; 8, least serious; and 12, no reported couvade symptoms. Of the 12 with serious cases, 11 had experienced stillbirths, twin births, and/or seriously abnormal births in prior pregnancies of the focal wife or other wives. The remaining case in this category (see Table I: case 9) was peculiar. In addition to the focal wife, who was suspected of pregnancy that turned out to be false, the man had had four other wives and children by none. Two wives had been divined as seriously, but temporarily barren and had been divorced some years earlier. Each divorced wife had remarried and now had one or more children, and both wives were again pregnant. This man was extremely anxious over the fact that he was childless despite many wives and years of trying. He claimed that the difficulty was due to witchcraft directed at him through his wives' temporary barrenness.[13] Ten of the men with serious cases had experienced extremely severe complications in prior pregnancies of the focal wife or other wives and childbirth fatalities of other wives. Eight had either no children or no male children by any wife. Of the 4 cases of fatalities of the focal wife in the present birth, 3 of the men exhibited serious symptoms. The other man (Table I: case 24), who had only least serious symptoms, was about to divorce the focal wife and seemed to care little about her or her childbearing capacity under the circumstances. In addition, the 8 men with serious cases in which there were no children or no male children included 5 of the 7 cases in which the fathers themselves were firstborn sons, and the 2 other men exhibited less (but not least) serious symptoms.

Of the 5 men with less serious symptoms, 2 had experienced stillbirths and/or serious abnormal births with prior pregnancies of some wife. There were no childbirth fatalities for any wife of these men, but 2 had experienced severe complications in prior pregnancies of the focal wife or other wives. Among these cases, 3 men had either no children or no male children, and 2 of these fathers were firstborn sons. Taking into account the firstborn status of the fathers, twin births, stillbirths, severely abnormal births, severe childbirth complications for wives, childbirth fatalities of wives, and either no children or no male children, the cases of serious symptoms exhibit an average of 4.17 such characteristics per case. In contrast, the men with less serious (1.00), least serious (1.00), and no symptoms (1.40) exhibited much lower frequencies of such traits.

In the wives of the 8 men with least serious symptoms, there were no stillbirths or severely abnormal births experienced. The single case (Table I: case 24) of a childbirth fatality of a wife was that of the man who was divorcing the woman who died. Among these cases, however, 2 men had experienced severe complications in prior pregnancies of the focal wife, but not of other wives. In contrast, for the most serious cases, 2 men had experienced such complications with both focal and other wives; 4, with only focal wives; and 4, with only other wives. For the less serious cases, none of the men had experienced severe complications with both focal and other wives; 1, with only a focal wife; and 1, with only another wife. In the men with no reported symptoms, none had experienced severe complications with both focal and other wives; 2, with only focal wives; and 2, with only other wives. Of the men with the least serious symptoms, 3 of the men had no children, but none had only female children. In contrast, of the men with serious symptoms, 4 had only daughters and 2 had no children. Of the men with less serious symptoms, 1 had only daughters and 2 had no children. Of the men with no reported symptoms, 2 had only daughters and 6 had no children. All of the men with the most serious symptoms had experienced some wife's prior pregnancy, with the anomalous instance of a false pregnancy in the case of the man who had tried and failed to have children with five wives (Table I: case 9). Of the 12 men with no prior experience of any wife's pregnancy, 2 exhibited less serious, 4 least serious, and 6 no reported symptoms.

In the wives of the 12 men with no reported symptoms there were no stillbirths, twin births, or severely abnormal births. Among these men, 4 had experienced severe complications in prior pregnancies of some wife but none had experienced a childbirth fatality of any wife. Of these fathers, 2 had no sons, but all of the 6 men who had no children also had never experienced a previous pregnancy of any wife. This category of cases is particularly difficult to assess insofar as *all* symptoms are reckoned entirely in terms of divination and formal presenting complaints and not of clinical examinations (except of the most naive, general, and observational variety with a few simple diagnostic measures). No doubt there may be some cultural self-fulfilling prophecy in these data by virtue of an exclusive reliance on Bimin-Kuskusmin modes of selection, categorization, and interpretation of symptoms and characterizations of critical indexes of vulnerability. Thus, the men with no symptoms may well ignore aspects of stress and disease that are not perceived through the cultural lens of couvade, and the culturally induced stress and emphasis of couvade may generate or exacerbate particular problems. Yet, if one is to explore the potential range of features of psychosomatic disorders, it is essential to examine the cultural construction of vulnerability and illness as a significant problem.

It is at least clear that Bimin-Kuskusmin recognize the key factors in the birth-related stress of fathers to be the following: (1) firstborn status of fathers; (2) no prior children or sons (but *with* prior experience of wives' pregnancies); and (3) traumatic prior experience of wives' childbearing (twin births, stillbirths, severely abnormal births, and childbirth complications and fatalities of wives). Divinatory diagnosis focuses on such factors, and both symptoms and classes of symptoms of varying degrees of severity are linked to these key factors. In turn, the severity of symptoms and classes of symptoms are linked to therapeutic alterations or strategic adjustments in the kind, degree, number, combination, and duration of couvade restrictions, and to the extent of couvade participation of the cognatic "therapy managing group." Bimin-Kuskusmin diagnosis is also sensitive, however, to the number, kind, degree, combination, and duration of couvade symptoms as well as to the severity of those symptoms and classes of symptoms. Furthermore, diagnostic attention is focused on whether or not particular symptoms or clusters of symptoms were present *before* the "sacred womb rite" and thus were only exacerbated by birth-related stress. For example, cases 4, 5, and 27 in Table I are the only instances in my sample in which bloody diarrhea and severe upper respiratory ailments were recognized as consequences *exclusively* of birth-related stress. These cases all involved fathers who were firstborn sons and who had prior experience of stillbirths, severely abnormal births, and childbirth complications and fatalities of wives. In other instances of these symptoms (cases 13 [stillbirth and childbirth complications] and 23 [severely abnormal birth, childbirth complications, and no sons] in Table I), there was evidence of prior amebic dysentery (case 13) or pneumonia (case 23); and the "same" symptoms were divined as being less serious in these cases because of non-birth-related causation than in the previously mentioned cases (cases 4, 5, and 27).

Given the apparent psychophysiological stress of couvade ritual itself, one might question the putative efficacy of "therapeutic" increases in these often harsh and debilitating observances. Bimin-Kuskusmin claim, however, that the relative severity of different phases of normal couvade observances *is* correlated with the relative debilitation of the father but that birth-related stress — unmodified by the special circumstances of particular fathers — follows a predictable pattern and the relative severity of couvade is a therapeutic response to, rather than a cause of, the consequent debilitation. In those men in whom no symptoms are noted, therefore, there is no special adjustment of couvade "therapy" beyond the cultural expectations of normal birth-related stress. In the cases of least serious symptoms, there is only minor adjustment of couvade ritual for therapeutic (either preventative or healing) purposes based on assessments of particular "case histories" and divinations. Although hardly conclusive, therefore, it may be suggestive to examine the cases of serious and less serious couvade symptoms. In these 17 cases, 113 symptoms – registered as presenting complaints and/or divinatory assessments – were recorded, with an average of 6.7 per case and a range of from 9 to 1 in any given case. The serious cases exhibited a range from 9 to 4 symptoms and an average of 8.0 per case, and the less serious cases exhibited a range from 7 to 1 and an average of 3.4 per case. All of these symptoms were judged to be relevant and legitimate vis-à-vis both general and specific patterns of birth-related stress in each case by means of various forms of social consensus that are bound up with couvade ritual. In the serious cases, after therapeutic intervention based on divination and consequent adjustment in the kind, degree, number, combination, and duration of couvade restrictions, 54 of the 96 symptoms were no longer either reported as presenting complaints or divined. In the less serious cases, after typically fewer, different, less intense, shorter, and less complex adjustments in couvade observances, 6 of the 17 symptoms were no longer either reported or divined. Thus, both presenting complaints and divinations do indicate for Bimin-Kuskusmin a positive efficacy of couvade ritual as a form of "therapy" through a recognized and marked decrease in the general and case-specific characteristics of the symptoms of birth-related stress.

There are many possible explanations for this traditionally recognized pattern of symptom reduction. Longitudinal case histories and clinical examinations of all "pregnant fathers" would be desirable but were not possible given the brevity of field research, my competence in clinical matters, and Bimin-Kuskusmin tolerance for this mode of inquiry. I should note, however, a few key characteristics of birth and couvade that may be relevant in this context. Bimin-Kuskusmin are acutely aware of the severe risks of childbearing, the probabilities of losing both wife and child, and the almost inevitable fatalities that follow any severe complications of childbirth. Similarly, the tragedies of stillbirths, twin births, and abnormal births are perceived as being more frequent than statistical assessments indicate. Many men have endured such traumas, and some of these men present empirically sensitive analyses of the features and apparent causes of birth-related misfortunes within their experience. Yet, pronounced anxiety is almost always present and most acute among those men who have had direct, personal experience of birth-related misfortunes within their own families or the families of close kin. Both delicate clinical interviews and several interrelated projective tests have been useful indexes of such birth-related stress and anxiety. Indeed, these several modes of probing particular "case histories" indicate quite consistent patterns of response to these misfortunes.

The loss of a wife or a child, especially when one has no others or no sons, is not only a personal tragedy but also a major social disability for a man, because the unmarried or childless man is often unable to achieve prominence in many of the prestigious spheres of male social life. The loss is often associated with guilt and shame over personal responsibility in the matter and fear of malevolent, preternatural forces and more mortal enmity. No doubt, substantial birth-related stress and anxiety may be identified, labeled, and shaped by cultural expectation, construction, legitimation, and expression of selected symptoms in couvade. Indeed, there is some evidence of social pressure toward symptomatically responding in appropriate ways to the formal and informal inquiries of couvade "diagnosis." Such culturally constituted signs of helplessness and vulnerability in crisis, however, are also a sanctioned demand for attention and ritual, social, and psychological support by significant others among one's kin, regardless of other strains in the tenor of relations with cognatic kin. In fact, social tensions among cognatic kin are abrogated by the formal requirements of couvade observances. In addition, the detailed traditional prescriptions and proscriptions of couvade that fall on both "pregnant fathers" and their kin and that are adjusted to the needs of the father by ritual authority and social consensus provide a concrete focus for both ritual and social recognition and support of birth-related stress and anxiety. Thus, for adult males involved in the life crisis of birth, couvade is a context in which diffuse, personal anxieties may be expressed openly and legitimately and in which ritual and social support provides public recognition of birth-related stress, empathy, and assurance that one's well-being is of central concern to a wide range of kin, who share in one's crisis and vulnerability.

Of particular interest is the fact that virtually *all* symptoms that are associated with couvade, when they are *not* linked to birth events, are brought to the attention of local Western clinics for treatment as much as any other symptoms of illness. Yet, when they appear as the symptoms of a "pregnant father," Western health care is adamantly avoided, as it is in all gynecological-obstetrical matters. This avoidance is of both theoretical interest and pragmatic concern, for the advantages of recently introduced Western biomedicine have no direct impact on birth-related disease or mortality among the Bimin-Kuskusmin.

BIRTH, CLINIC, AND BIMIN-KUSKUSMIN SKEPTICISM

Among the several Western medical facilities that are available in some manner to Bimin-Kuskusmin, the clinic of the Australian Baptist Missionary Society to the north among the Tekin Oksapmin people is the only one to offer gynecological-obstetrical services. This clinic, staffed by Oksapmin women under the supervision of a trained European nurse, shows considerable interest in pregnant women and newborn infants and encourages local people to attend its "baby patrols" and to give birth within its complex. Yet, by 1973, no known Bimin-Kuskusmin birth had occurred at the mission clinic, nor had any pregnant Bimin-Kuskusmin woman or new mother sought medical assistance there or from the clinic's traveling medical patrols. Based on their own perceptions of the beliefs and practices of this clinic, Bimin-Kuskusmin give several reasons for their utter avoidance of its services in contexts of pregnancy and birth.

First, typical clinical examinations are considered to be not only a serious breach of etiquette but also a special danger in contexts of pregnancy and birth. The use of a general anesthetic precludes the consciousness of the mother at a critical time when she must exert active control in childbearing and must respond alertly to the instructions and inquiries of the midwife. To divulge the intimacies of personal "case histories" beyond the secure sphere of close cognatic kin and healer-diviners is to invite mortal harm in many ways. To permit the probing of bodily parts and orifices is to suffer great humiliation and to expose oneself and one's child to injury through witchcraft and other nefarious means. The taking of samples of bodily substances, the administration of unknown medicines, and the incomprehensible alterations of diet are especially feared. Bimin-Kuskusmin feel strongly that the critical and delicate balances of "male" and "female" substances, which are shaped, controlled, nurtured, or altered in accordance with the couvade "model of therapy," are destroyed or damaged by such bodily intrusions and that they cannot ritually remedy such uncomprehended acts. Even the ritually important placenta and umbilical cord are discarded in the mission birth clinic. The Bimin-Kuskusmin are convinced that such clinical practices provoke mortal illness or barrenness, and they cite the absence of unadopted European children at the mission as a most suspicious omen. Furthermore, the clinic staff that controls administration of medicine and diet, and that has ready access to specimens of bodily substance taken in examination, are Tekin Oksapmin women, who are from a hostile ethnic group and represent the origin of the feared and lethal *tamam* witchcraft (Poole, 1981b). Poisoning and witchcraft and sorcery act most efficiently through ingested or detached foods and bodily substances. The Tekin Oksapmin have both the techniques and the motives, as well as the means in the context of the clinic, to inflict mortal harm, and the Bimin-Kuskusmin who are centrally involved in birth events are particularly vulnerable to their malevolent onslaughts.

Second, the mission personnel are not only beyond the pale of Bimin-Kuskusmin social control but also otherwise inappropriate for the practice of midwifery. The clinic staff of Tekin Oksapmin females are young and unmarried and often uninitiated as adult women, and they have no personal experience of childbearing. They not only carry the potential for wielding lethal witchcraft but also are unrelated to any Bimin-Kuskusmin by kinship or marriage and thus are beyond the range of jural, moral, political, and ritual control. No traditional sanctions can be brought to bear effectively on their behavior, and they are believed to harbor intense hatred for all Bimin-Kuskusmin who are their traditional enemies. Furthermore, the Tekin Oksapmin are said to have very high childbirth mortality and chronically sick children as a consequence of both bizarre and dangerous birth practices and rampant witchcraft, and they practice no analog of the Bimin-Kuskusmin "sacred womb rite." In turn, the European nurse, who is of the appropriate age and postmenopausal status for a midwife, is said never to have been married, to have no children or personal experience of childbearing, and to have no known kin in the area, all of which are minimal prerequisites of becoming a Bimin-Kuskusmin midwife. The efficacy of her apparent ritual knowledge and skills is unknown. She is not only beyond the range of Bimin-Kuskusmin social control but also is known to be highly dogmatic and authoritarian in matters of conception, pregnancy, childbirth, postpartum events, and related clinical examinations. Finally, she is said to dismiss local traditions concerning birth-related belief and practice in the course of intense proselytization of mission belief and practice, which is often seen as antithetical to Bimin-Kuskusmin custom.

Third, the clinic is widely known to be intolerant of traditional beliefs and practices associated with traditional religion and to proselytize in all ostensibly medical contexts. Since Bimin-Kuskusmin too draw no consistent conceptual distinction between matters of "medicine" and "religion," they do not fault mission proselytization per se. They do fear the consequences of the mission approach, however, for traditional ritual performances and ancestral intervention are believed to be utterly central to childbearing. Ancestors are invoked in many divinations that are used to monitor the essential balances of "male" and "female" substances that must be maintained throughout normal pregnancy and birth and under the variable circumstances of birth-related stress and anxiety. The "therapy" of couvade requires the use of certain ritual *sacrae* and the activity of certain ritual personnel that are excluded from the mission during both pregnancy and birth. Bimin-Kuskusmin find an intolerable arrogance in proselytization of this kind, and such an affront to their own ritual traditions is thought to be most dangerous in the context of the life crises of pregnancy, birth, and parenthood.

Finally, and most important with respect to couvade, Bimin-Kuskusmin fear the mission's unyielding exclusion of all people at risk or otherwise critically involved in childbearing events except the mother and child, who together seem to constitute the exclusive social fabric of birth from the clinic's perspective. The pregnant woman is utterly isolated from her kin, affines, and ritual experts, who are forbidden to visit her. Yet, she is placed in intimate contact with dangerous, alien women who are believed to be witches. At the birth of a child, mother and infant are inexplicably separated on numerous occasions and the fragile baby is examined and fondled by utter strangers and is fed liquids other than the mother's breast milk. All cognatic kin of the father, mother, and child, as well as the clan midwife and the "pregnant father," are denied access to the maternity ward despite their protestations. Thus, the mother and child are excluded from all advice, divination, social support, and ritual control of the tradition of couvade. In turn, without the ability to observe and to monitor delicately the course of late pregnancy and birth, the midwife, the "pregnant father," and the cognatic kin of both parents and child cannot properly plan or coordinate couvade observances outside the mission complex. Thus, *all* participants in Bimin-Kuskusmin birth events and couvade ritual and "therapy," particularly the father, mother, and child, are left in a position of severe and enduring risk in a threatening environment and without any semblance of traditional protection against stress, anxiety, and illness, or of essential ritual, social, and psychological support.

In this precarious situation, the position of the "pregnant father" is seen to be particularly disturbing, for his acute vulnerability to birth-related stress and illness as a father is generally ignored by the mission clinic. There is a critical contrast here between Bimin-Kuskusmin and mission understandings of the position of the father in life crises of birth. On the one hand, the presenting complaints of new fathers tend to be translated by the clinic into the symptoms of a diversity of diseases that are reckoned in Western biomedical terms. Such symptoms are perceived by the clinic as being entirely unrelated to the course of pregnancy, birth, and postpartum events, in which the father is intimately involved, by Bimin-Kuskusmin reckoning, in terms of bonds of substance and spirit and in terms of affective and social participation. There is no notion of potentially birth-related ailments of males in the mission's repertoire of diagnostic categories. Thus, the Bimin-Kuskusmin reasonably suspect that the clinic cannot successfully treat what it cannot properly diagnose. Palliative treatment of isolated or improperly clustered symptoms is insufficient, for the etiological reckoning of illness is defective. Vulnerable persons remain at risk, and perhaps the risk increases due to the dangerous peculiarities of Western clinical treatment and clinicians. On the other hand, the presenting complaints of new fathers are held to be distinctively birth-related illness phenomena by the Bimin-Kuskusmin, and they are diagnosed and managed therapeutically by delicate adjustments in the symbolic and social dimensions of couvade that are based on equally sensitive assessments of the etiology of the father's vulnerability to stress and illness in life crises of birth. Thus, couvade symptoms are recognized as indexes of both general and particular birth-related illnesses, and couvade ritual provides a cultural model of (cognitively) and for (therapeutically) such illnesses.

In consequence, the Bimin-Kuskusmin entirely avoid the mission clinic in all birth-related matters. In some ways, this negative reaction of both the Bimin-Kuskusmin and the mission clinic to each other's traditions concerning birth events is a tragedy. There are aspects of Bimin-Kuskusmin beliefs and practices concerning pregnancy, childbirth, and postpartum events that are certainly ineffective or even detrimental by Western biomedical standards and that would benefit from a more sensitive introduction of Western gynecological and obstetrical insights than they have experienced. In turn, the often subtle psychological, social, and behavioral insights of the Bimin-Kuskusmin cultural model of couvade ritual are worthy of close scrutiny and perhaps some delicate cross-cultural translation by advocates of a more biomedical model of the significant stresses and vulnerabilities of pregnancy, birth, and postpartum events.

CONCLUSION

This chapter has explored some of the ways in which a remote Papua New Guinea people conceptualize the interrelationships between pregnancy, birth, and postpartum events, on the one hand, and birth-related vulnerability, stress, illness, ritual, therapy, and social and psychological support, on the other. An elaborate cultural focus on the "pregnant father" is central to the Bimin-Kuskusmin "sacred womb rite." By examining critical linkages between couvade symptoms and couvade ritual, I have examined a detailed ethnographical example of how an apparent diversity of psychophysiological disturbances in men who are involved in birth events may be recognized, evaluated, labeled, and managed as illness through encompassment by a ritual of birth. In the West, where couvade ritual is extremely rare, "couvade syndrome" (Trethowan, 1972) is most difficult to diagnose or otherwise assess with certainty since neither folk nor biomedical etiological categories are available for diagnosis, prognosis, and treatment. As in the case of the mission clinic among the Bimin-Kuskusmin, male symptoms at times of life crises of birth are often "read" as indexes of diseases that do not include birth-related stresses among their critical features. Thus, such symptoms are often perceived as being etiologically diverse and thus are subject to diverse diagnostic classifications and treatments.

As Lipkin and Lamb note in Chapter 6, the characteristics of a man's presenting complaints during a wife's pregnancy and child-bearing are often variable and seemingly idiosyncratic in ways that make diagnosis of a consistent "couvade syndrome" difficult and challenging. There is neither a cultural illness nor a biomedical disease model available in any unambiguous way. By contrast, the Bimin-Kuskusmin case illustrates how a cultural model of birth-related vulnerability, stress, anxiety, and illness recognizes, labels, treats, and even shapes individual vulnerabilities and symptoms so that they can be diagnosed and managed as illnesses within a particular etiological framework. Yet, each case presents its own dilemma. On the one hand, the Western biomedical model is well adapted to dealing with male symptoms at times of birth events as being significant indexes of non-birth-related disease categories, but it is less attuned to recognizing at least some of these symptoms as indexes of a birth-related category of disease. On the other hand, the Bimin-Kuskusmin couvade model tends to collapse most of the symptoms of "pregnant fathers" into a single category of birth-related illnesses and largely to ignore other possibilities of illnesses that can co-occur with couvade illnesses. The contrast suggests that greater cultural, psychological, and social sensitivity in the introduction of Western health care is essential. Attention to cultural notions of stress and illness will not only facilitate this introduction of Western concepts and practices in a useful manner to other non-Western societies but also will enhance the sensitivity of the Western biomedical model itself to the full range of intertwined dimensions of human suffering (cf. Kleinman, Eisenberg, and Good, 1978). To the extent that folk and biomedical models become more sensitive to each other's concerns, the threat of inappropriate medicalization that violates the cultural, psychological, and social needs of people must become less severe and at least recognizable as a problem.

NOTES

1. For example, the Boston Women's Health Book Collective suggests that, "Home birth offers a woman the opportunity to labor in familiar surroundings; to choose her own attendants; to follow rituals and actions which soothe and encourage her. At home she avoids the annoying, and sometimes dangerous, hospital routines. At home, birth is a family event . . ." (1976, p. 269).
2. The data for this analysis are drawn from field research among the Bimin-Kuskusmin from 1971 to 1973. Research was generously supported by the U.S. National Institutes of Health, the Cornell University Humanities and Social Sciences Program, and the Center for South Pacific Studies of the

University of California, Santa Cruz. The New Guinea Research Unit of the Australian National University provided valuable assistance. The Bimin-Kuskusmin people, for sharing the joy and the trauma of birth, are owed the primary debt of gratitude. For thoughtful commentary on an earlier draft of this essay, I thank M. de Vries, G. Harris, J. Janzen, A. Kleinman, G. Lewis, M. Lipkin, J. H. Pfifferling, W. Sangree, and H. J. Simon. Final responsibility for the published version is, of course, my own.

3. The notion of "couvade ritual phenomena" bears some affinity to related ideas of "ritual couvade" (Trethowan, 1965, 1968, 1972; Trethowan and Conlon, 1965) and "social couvade" (Newman, 1966), which emphasize the customary or socioculturally articulated phenomena of anthropological concern.

4. The notion of "variable psychophysiological couvade symptoms" bears some affinity to related ideas of "couvade syndrome" (Trethowan, 1965, 1968, 1972; Trethowan and Conlon, 1965), *Mitleiden* (Polgar, 1963), and "psychosomatic couvade" (Newman, 1966), which emphasize phenomena of psychiatric concern. For related analytical distinctions, see also Kupferer, 1965; Munroe and Munroe, 1971, 1973; Munroe, Munroe, and Nerlove, 1973; and Munroe, Munroe, and Whiting, 1965, 1973.

5. The analytic distinction between "illness" and "disease" is drawn from the valuable insights of Fabrega (1974, 1975, 1977) and Kleinman (1973, 1974-75, 1978). See also Engel's (1977) significant contribution in this regard.

6. The *finiik* spirit, which is procreatively transmitted patrilineally through semen, represents the ordered and controlled jural and moral aspects of the person. It contrasts with the *khaapkhabuurien* spirit, which represents the more idiosyncratic, private self and the distinguishing characteristics of the individual actor.

7. Due to complex ideas concerning the procreative transmissions of "agnatic blood" through both men and women (albeit in a more restricted manner; see Poole, 1981c), a cognatic kindred extends beyond a parent's lineage to the lineages of the parent's mother, father's mother, mother's mother, father's father's mother, father's mother's mother, mother's father's mother, and mother's mother's mother. A parent will share with a child, however, the "agnatic blood" of only his or her own lineage and the lineages of his or her mother, father's mother, and mother's mother.

8. The irregularity of Bimin-Kuskusmin menstrual cycles after adolescent sterility following first menses at 17 to 18 years of age may be due, in part, to a generally protein-deficient diet, sporadic bouts of severe famine, and abruptly shifting constellations of food taboos throughout the female life cycle, as well as frequent and chronic parasitical problems and other intestinal ailments.

9. For males, sexual intercourse is always debilitating and is said to account for many illnesses and premature signs of aging, but the excessive loss of semen during the frequent intercourse during a wife's pregnancy, which is accompanied by other aspects of couvade stress, is the most debilitating of all forms except for lethal intercourse with *tamam* witches (Poole, 1981b).

10. Distant, nonparticipating cognatic kin are dangerous to birth events and proper couvade performances because they are potentially witches, who can launch attacks on father, mother, and child only through cognatic (especially uterine) links. The fact that such kin are not participating in couvade and are thus ignoring significant jural and moral obligations marks them as potential witches.

11. White pigment symbolizes in the context of couvade both the masculine force and power of bone, semen, and taro and the feminine quality of nurturance and fertility associated with the umbilical cord and the "fertile fluids" (*mem gom*). White often contrasts to red, which symbolizes the male qualities of "agnatic blood" and patrilineal connections, and black, which symbolizes the female evils of menstrual blood, uterine connections, illness, death, and witchcraft. In this particular context, the mixture of white pigment and sow fat, however, signifies a primarily "female" protective shield against particularly "black blood illnesses," female spirits, and witches.

12. Bimin-Kuskusmin recognize the demographic fact that infant mortality tends to be highest between birth and the appearance of deciduous teeth, when "female names" are given. There is considerable anxiety expressed by most parents over the health of the infant during this exceptionally vulnerable period of approximately the first two years of life.

13. Male sterility is not recognized as a "natural" possibility among the Bimin-Kuskusmin. In contrast, female barrenness is a matter of much concern, elaborate divinatory diagnosis, and in many cases of therapeutic intervention through ritual performances involving the ingestion of fertility substances.

REFERENCES

Ayres, B. 1967. Pregnancy Magic: A Study of Food Taboos and Sex Avoidances. In *Cross-Cultural Approaches*, ed. C. S. Ford, pp. 111-25. New Haven: HRAF Press.

Bachofen, J. J. 1861. *Das Mutterrecht*. Basel, Benno Schwabe.

Bettelheim, B. 1962. *Symbolic Wounds*. New York: Collier Books.

Blackwood, B. 1935. *Both Sides of Buka Passage*. Oxford: Clarendon Press.

Boston Women's Health Book Collective. 1976. *Our Bodies, Our Selves*. New York: Simon and Schuster.

Briffault, R. 1931. Birth Customs. *Encyclopaedia Soc. Sci.* 2:565-66.

Cavenar, J., and Butts, N. 1977. Fatherhood and Emotional Illness. *Am. J. Psychiatry* 134:429-32.

Coelho, R. 1949. The Significance of Couvade among the Black Caribs. *Man* 49:51-53.

Coleman, A. D., and Coleman, L. L. 1971. The Expectant Father's Experience. In *Pregnancy*, ed. A. D. Coleman and L. L. Coleman, pp. 96-143. New York: Seabury Press.

Colson, A. B. 1975. Birth Customs of the Akawaio. In *Studies in Social Anthropology*, ed. J. H. M. Beattie and R. G. Lienhardt, pp. 285-309. Oxford: Clarendon Press.

Corso, R. 1953-54. La "Couvade" y su Interpretación. *Runa* 6:133-41.

Crawley, E. 1960. *The Mystic Rose*. New York: Meridian Books.

Curtis, J. 1955. A Psychiatric Study of 55 Expectant Fathers. *U.S. Armed Forces Med. J.* 6:937-50.

Da Matta, R. 1971. O Sistema Relações Apinayé: Terminologia e Ideologia. Rio de Janeiro: Museu Nacional of the Federal University of Rio de Janeiro. Mimeographed.

Dawson, W. R. 1929. *The Custom of Couvade*. Manchester: Manchester University Press.

de Josselin de Jong, J. P. B. 1922. De Couvade. *Mededeelingen der Koninklijke Akademie van Wetenschappen, Afdeling Letterkunde* 54(B):53-84.

Diaz, M. N. 1965. Scandinavian Birth Customs. Santa Cruz: University of California, Santa Cruz. Mimeographed.

Douglas, M. 1975. Couvade and Menstruation: The Relevance of Tribal Studies. In *Implicit Meanings*, ed. M. Douglas, pp. 60-72. London: Routledge and Kegan Paul.

Driver, H. E. 1969. Couvade. *Encyclopaedia Britannica* 6:674.

Dumont, L. 1972. Une Science en Devenir. *L'Arc* 48:8-21.

Engel, G. L. 1977. The Need for a New Medical Model: A Challenge for Biomedicine. *Science* 196:129-36.

Evans, W. N. 1951. Simulated Pregnancy in a Male. *Psychoanal. Q.* 20:165-78.

Fabrega, H., Jr. 1974. *Disease and Social Behavior*. Cambridge, Mass.: M.I.T. Press.

_____. 1975. The Need for an Ethnomedical Science. *Science* 189:969-75.

_____. 1977. The Scope of Ethnomedical Science. *Culture Med. Psychiatry* 1:201-28.

Fock, N. 1967. South American Birth Customs in Theory and Practice. In *Cross-Cultural Approaches*, ed. C. S. Ford, pp. 126-44. New Haven: HRAF Press.

Fortes, M. 1973. On the Concept of the Person among the Tallensi. In *La Notion de Personne en Afrique Noire*, ed. G. Dieterlen, pp. 283-319. Paris: Editions du Centre National de la Recherche Scientifique.

_____. 1974. The First Born. *J. Child Psychol. Psychiatry* 15:81-104.

_____. 1978. The Significance of the First Born in African Family Systems. In *Systèmes de Signes*, ed. Centre National de la Recherche Scientifique, pp. 131-50. Paris: Hermann.

Fox, R. 1977. The Medicalization and Demedicalization of American Society. *Daedalus* (Winter 1977):9-22.

Frazer, J. G. 1910. *Totemism and Exogamy*. London: Macmillan.

Freeman, T. 1951. Pregnancy as a Precipitant of Mental Illness in Men. *Brit. J. Med. Psychol.* 24:49-54.

Freud, S. 1942. *Collected Papers of Sigmund Freud*, Vol. 2, ed. E. Jones. London: Institute of Psychoanalysis.

Ginath, Y. 1974. Psychoses in Males in Relation to Their Wives' Pregnancy and Childbirth. *Isr. Ann. Psychiatry* 12:228-37.

Glick, L. B. 1963. Foundations of a Primitive Medical System. Ph.D. dissertation, University of Pennsylvania.

Gurwitt, A. 1976. Aspects of Prospective Fatherhood: A Case Report. *Psychoanal. Study Child* 31:237-72.

Harris, G. G. 1978. *Casting out Anger.* London: Cambridge University Press.

Hayano, D. M. 1974. Misfortune and Traditional Political Leadership among the Tauna Awa of New Guinea. *Oceania* 45:18-26.

Hiatt, L. R. 1971. Secret Pseudo-Procreative Rites among the Australian Aborigines. In *Anthropology in Oceania*, ed. L. R. Hiatt and C. Jayawardena, pp. 77-88. Sydney: Angus and Robertson.

Hogbin, H. I. 1943. A New Guinea Infancy: From Conception to Weaning in Wogeo. *Oceania* 13:285-309.

——. 1970. *The Island of Menstruating Men.* Scranton: Chandler Publishing.

Hogenboom, P. 1967. Man in Crisis: The Father. *J. Psychiatric Nursing* 5:457-64.

Hott, J. 1976. The Crisis of Expectant Fatherhood. *Am. J. Nursing* 76:1436-40.

Illich, I. 1976. *Medical Nemesis: The Expropriation of Health.* New York: Pantheon Books.

Jaffe, D. 1968. Masculine Envy of Women's Procreative Function. *J. Am. Psychoanal. Assoc.* 16:521-48.

Janzen, J. M. 1978. The Comparative Study of Medical Systems as Changing Social Systems. *Soc. Sci. Med.* 12(B):121-29.

Jarvis, W. 1962. Some Effects of Pregnancy and Childbirth on Men. *J. Am. Psychoanal. Assoc.* 10:689-99.

Josselyn, I. 1956. Cultural Forces, Motherliness and Fatherliness. *Am. J. Orthopsychiatry* 26:264-71.

Karsten, R. 1915. The Couvade or Male Child-bed among the South American Indians. *Öfversikt af Finska Vetenskaps-Societetens Förhandlingar* 57:1914-15.

King, E. 1968. The Pregnant Father. *Bull. Am. Coll. Nurse-Midwifery* 13:19-25.

Kleinman, A. M. 1973. Medicine's Symbolic Reality: On a Central Problem in the Philosophy of Medicine. *Inquiry* 16:206-13.

——. 1974-75. Cognitive Structures of Traditional Medical Systems: Ordering, Explaining, and Interpreting the Human Experience of Illness. *Ethnomedicine* 3:27-49.

——. 1978. Concepts and a Model for the Comparison of Medical Systems as Cultural Systems. *Soc. Sci. Med.* 12(B):85-93.

Kleinman, A. M.; Eisenberg, L.; and Good, B. 1978. Culture, Illness and Care: Clinical Lessons from Anthropological and Cross-Cultural Research. *Ann. Intern. Med.* 88:251-58.

Kroeber, A. L. 1948. *Anthropology.* New York: Harcourt, Brace and World.

Kupferer, H. J. K. 1965. Couvade: Ritual or Real Illness. *Am. Anthropologist* 67:99-102.

Lévi-Strauss, C. 1962. *La Pensée Sauvage.* Paris: Plon.

Malinowski, B. 1927. *Sex and Repression in Savage Society.* New York: Harcourt, Brace.

Mead, M. 1970. *The Mountain Arapesh II.* Garden City, N.J.: Natural History Press.

Meigs, A. S. 1976. Male Pregnancy and the Reduction of Sexual Opposition in a New Guinea Highlands Society. *Ethnology* 15:393-407.

Métraux, A. 1963. The Couvade. In *Handbook of South American Indians*, Vol. 5, ed. J. H. Steward, pp. 369-74. New York: Cooper Square Publishers.

Munroe, R. L., and Munroe, R. H. 1971. Male Pregnancy Symptoms and Cross-Sex Identity in Three Societies. *J. Soc. Psychol.* 84:11-25.

———. 1973. Psychological Interpretation of Male Initiation Rites: The Case of Male Pregnancy Symptoms. *Ethos* 1:490-98.

Munroe, R. L.; Munroe, R. H.; and Nerlove, S. B. 1973. Male Pregnancy Symptoms and Cross-Sex Identity: Two Replications. *J. Soc. Psychol.* 89:147-48.

Munroe, R. L.; Munroe, R. H.; and Whiting, J. W. M. 1965. Structure and Sentiment: Evidence from Recent Studies of the Couvade. Denver: Annual Meeting of the American Anthropological Association. Mimeographed.

———. 1973. The Couvade: A Psychological Analysis. *Ethos* 1:30-74.

Newman, L. 1966. The Couvade: A Reply to Kupferer. *Am. Anthropologist* 153-56.

Obrzut, L. 1976. Expectant Fathers' Perception of Fathering. *Am. J. Nursing* 76:1440-42.

Paige, K. E., and Paige, J. M. 1981. *The Politics of Reproductive Ritual*. Berkeley: University of California Press.

Ploss, H. 1911. *Das Kind in Brauch und Sitte der Völker*. Leipzig: Grieben.

Polgar, S. 1963. Parental Emotions in Pregnancy. Chapel Hill: University of North Carolina. Mimeographed.

Poole, F. J. P. 1976a. "Knowledge Rests in the Heart": Bimin-Kuskusmin Metacommunications on Meaning, Tacit Knowledge, and Field Research. Washington, D.C.: Annual Meeting of the American Anthropological Association. Mimeographed.

———. 1976b. The *Ais Am*. Ph.D. dissertation, Cornell University.

———. 1981a. Cultural Significance of "Drunken Comportment" in a Non-Drinking Society: The Case of the Bimin-Kuskusmin of Papua New Guinea. In *Alcohol Use and Abuse in Papua New Guinea*, ed. M. Marshall. Boroko: Papua New Guinea Institute of Applied Social and Economic Research.

———. 1981b. *Tamam*: Ideological and Sociological Configurations of "Witchcraft" among Bimin-Kuskusmin. *Soc. Anal.* in press.

———. 1981c. Transforming "Natural" Woman: Female Ritual Leaders and Gender Ideology among Bimin-Kuskusmin. In *Sexual Meanings*, ed. S. B. Ortner and H. Whitehead, pp. 116-65. London: Cambridge University Press.

Pospisil. L. 1978. *The Kapauku Papuans of West New Guinea*, 2nd ed. New York: Holt, Rinehart and Winston.

Powdermaker, H. 1971. *Life in Lesu*. New York: Norton.

Reik, T. 1931. *Ritual*, Trans. D. Bryan. New York: Norton.

Rivière, P. G. 1974. The Couvade: A Problem Reborn. *Man* (N.S.) 9:423-35.

Roth, H. L. 1893. On the Significance of the Couvade. *J. R. Anthropol. Inst.* 22:204-43.

Rubel, A., and Spielberg, J. 1966. Aspects of the Couvade in Texas and Northeast Mexico. In *Summa Antropológia en Homenaje a Roberto J. Weitlaner*, ed. Instituto Nacional de Antropología e Historia, pp. 299-307. Mexico City: Instituto Nacional de Antropología e Historia.

Schmidt, W. 1954. Gebräuche des Ehemannes bei Schwangerschaft und Geburt, mit Richtigstellung des Begriffes der Couvade. *Wien. Beitr. Kulturgeschichte Linguistik* 10:98-120.

Sedgwick, P. 1973. Illness, Mental and Otherwise: All Illnesses Express a Social Judgment. *Hastings Center Studies* 1(3):19-40.

Spencer, R. F. 1949-50. Primitive Obstetrics. *Ciba Symposium* 11:1158-88.

Trethowan, W. H. 1965. Sympathy Pains. *Discovery* 26:30-33.

——. 1968. The Couvade Syndrome — Some Further Observations. *J. Psychosom. Res.* 12:107-15.

——. 1972. The Couvade Syndrome. In *Modern Perspectives in Psycho-Obstetrics*, ed. J. Howells, pp. 68-93. Edinburgh: Oliver and Boyd.

Trethowan, W. H., and Conlon, M. F. 1965. The Couvade Syndrome. *Brit. J. Psychiatry* 111:57-66.

Tylor, E. B. 1865. *Researches into the Early History of Mankind and the Development of Civilization*. London: John Murray.

——. 1889. On a Method of Investigating the Development of Institutions: Applied to Laws of Marriage and Descent. *J. R. Anthropol. Inst.* 18:245-72.

——. 1892a. "Couvade" — The Genesis of an Anthropological Term. *The Academy* 1070:412.

——. 1892b. "Couvade" — The Genesis of an Anthropological Term. *The Academy* 1075:542.

van Gennep, A. 1909. *Les Rites de Passage*. Paris: Nourry.

Voegelin, C. F. 1960. Pregnancy Couvade Attested by Term and Text in Hopi. *Am. Anthropologist* 62:491-93.

Wainwright, W. 1968. Fatherhood as a Precipitant of Mental Illness. *Am. J. Psychiatry* 123: 40-44.

Young, F. W. 1965. *Initiation Ceremonies*. Indianapolis: Bobbs-Merrill.

Young, F. W., and Bacdayan, A. 1965. Menstrual Taboos and Social Rigidity. *Ethnology* 4:225-40.

6

COUVADE SYMPTOMS IN
A PRIMARY CARE PRACTICE:
Use of an Illness Without a Disease
to Examine Health Care Behavior

Mack Lipkin, Jr.
Gerri S. Lamb

This chapter was written to further understanding of a troublesome interface between medicine and people, the area of illness without palpable or externally (to the patient) measurable physical pathology. We are referring to those conditions in which the patient experiences physical distress but the physician (or other diagnostician) not only fails to find a physical lesion but does find (or theoretically could) reason for distress in another domain, such as the psychological or social context of the patient.

There are many objections to such inquiry. Steadfast reductionists argue that every situation causing distress has a physical substrate that could, theoretically, be measured. That may be a comforting theory with heuristic value. But it is a nonfalsifiable theory. It is of little or no use to those of us who practice in this century. If a healer chooses to respond as helpfully as possible to patients with pain and suffering, the high prevalence of mind-body problems is inescapable. Checking to see if such cases occur, how often they do, and what happens when they do also raises questions about what should be done about such cases.

That, of course, raises the central issue of medicalization arguments — what are medicine's functions? Is medicine merely to diagnose through physical measurement or other "proven" quasi-equivalents such as taking a history? Is it to report to the patient concerning the statistical probabilities of alteration of physical states through physical means (medical treatment), negotiate such an alteration, and execute it? Is it to attempt to understand and help the patient with those of their problems that they choose to bring to us and with which we feel competent to help. In this alternative, patients sort through their problems and present some for consideration. We use assessment techniques of several sorts, such as talking, feeling, being biased, and using objective testing, to decide which are assessable by us, which can be helped or comforted, and which are problems outside our domain. We even make decisions about what are problems and what are not. How do such decisions get made and on what basis?

Numerous constructs exist to cover this ground, such as tradition (Janzen, Chapter 1), scientific proof (Feinstein, 1967), role-related behavior (Parsons, 1951; Mechanic, 1961), the art of medicine (in our culture), and the role of the healer (in cultures studied by anthropologists) (Knowles, 1977).

We undertook a pilot study to try to develop an analytical tool to begin to analyze issues of psychosociogenic illness by using a clinical epidemiological method, the tracer method, with a common practice problem, in a large prepaid group practice treating a typical United States urban population (Lipkin and Lamb, 1982). We plan here to present the phenomenon we looked at, the couvade condition, and some of the other reasons it is of interest. Later, Lipkin writes of some of the relations of such events and medical problems, labels, and actions (see Chapter 9).

Our perspective in undertaking this work was that of a primary care internist and nurse practitioner concerned with the study of the nature of medical practice and the large portion (estimates vary widely [Regier, 1979; Hoeper, 1979; Schlesinger et al., 1979]) of practice concerned with psychogenic and social events. As practitioners, we are forced to deal with the complexities that real people bring. We came to notice quickly on starting clinical work that medical practitioners in this society encounter and ignore a large variety of phenomena for which their patients come to them for help. Each class of practitioners tends to apply a separate orientation, a separate set of paradigms, and a separate set of behaviors. Each asks stereotypical series of questions that lead to a limited variety of possible answers, examinations, explanations, behaviors, and outcomes.

In many cases the end result for the patient is a function of the chance that determines which channel of care is sought or entered.

Thus a patient with low back pain may get a urinalysis from a nephrologist, a pelvic examination from a gynecologist, a low back radiograph from an orthopedist, and a discussion of stress and life problems from a psychiatrist.

In our setting, a prepaid group practice with 36,000 members that is demographically typical of the working population of Rochester, New York (Wersinger and Roberts, 1977), approximately 4 percent of our patients present with problems for which no specific anatomical or pathophysiological diagnosis seems appropriate, even after specialist evaluations (Lipkin et al., 1977). They suffer, hurt, and demand help and so require both routine physical care and the services of a person able to recognize the existence of psychogenic illness, symbolic illness, or a complex interaction between concomitant disease and psychosomatic phenomena such as conversion.

It is fascinating to see how these patients (some 1,200) are managed when they are not recognized, as is usually the case. They get treated in the diagnostic style to which their physician has become accustomed: usually they are subjected to an extensive, expensive, sometimes invasive set of studies and sometimes experimental pharmacotherapeutic trials for a variety of nonspecific diagnostic catch-alls. For the gastrointestinal tract, these include such categories as peptic ulcer syndrome in the absence of definitive findings. For chest pain, labels of atypical angina, coronary spasm, or "ASCVD" get placed on them; they get angiograms, echocardiograms, stress tests, propranolol, diazepam, disability, and low cholesterol diets. For neck pain they get labeled variously, with older patients most often told they have degenerative arthritis and then getting braced, stretched, manipulated, and stuck on long term aspirin therapy. This is not to argue that these labels, diagnoses, and treatments are not sometimes helpful and corresponding to objective disease states. Rather it is to suggest that the uses of such labels extends into the gray areas of diagnosis in which the data do not always justify a discrete diagnosis either because the phenomena are nonspecific, are normal variants, are fictitious, or are nonfalsifiable. Here the issue is not of too much or too little medicalization. It is of sufficiently cogent, appropriate, and effective care based on sufficiently comprehensive models of health and illness.

A central aspect of our arguments will be that effective care depends on appropriate labeling and diagnosis and that the domains of diganosis are broader than current practice reflects. Indeed, in one new volume an international group argues that classification of health problems should now be broadened and changed from a single axis, monoetiological system to a triaxial system that reflects the interaction of physical, social, and psychological components of health problems (Lipkin and Kupka, 1982).

We undertook to provide an analytical tool for examining the incidence and prevalence of one psychosociogenic problem in our typical medical practice. By examining a psychosociogenic problem in which the question of concomitant disease and its complex interactions with symbolic illness was controlled, we hoped it might be possible to learn something about the methods used by medical care personnel to deal (or fail to deal) with a specific illness phenomenon. The problem we choose, couvade phenomenon, is defined as the occurrence in the mate of an expectant woman of (specified) pregnancylike or associated symptoms not previously or subsequently affecting the man nor otherwise objectively explained. Couvade is, in itself, intrinsically fascinating because of the complex issues it raises concerning sexual identity, the nature of subjective physical experience, and the relationship between one's development and ways of experiencing one's self physically and culturally.

The problem is also of interest because it is a major subject of anthropological research in which magnificent cross-cultural evaluations have been used to support theories about the nature of culture and the interaction of psychological ontogenesis and the development of cultural and personal events such as couvade symptoms and couvade ritual (Munroe and Munroe, 1971).

It was hoped that the use of an analytical tool such as the examination of an illness without a concomitant disease would provide new insights into the cultural and social roles of the physician and of the patient and how each of these influences the other's behavior. For the present purposes, we are using "illness" to denote the subjective state of discomfort in the body that is associated with seeking of medical care. We are using "disease" to denote the presence in a person of externally (what is usually meant by "objectively") detectable pathology or other physical abnormality associated with seeking or receiving medical care. The purpose of distinguishing these is to look at those cases in which the former exists without the latter. The present example of couvade alone is sufficient to warrant this distinction, although there are many other equally sufficient examples. Prior studies of these sorts of problems, and of couvade itself, have been somewhat muddied by lack of a clear example and by the confusion arising from the difficulty of sorting the psychogenic or sociogenic from the pathophysiological aspects of an illness-disease process. By far, the most common cases are those in which the two aspects are intermixed such as the older woman with new chest pains, nonspecific electrocardiographic changes, and a husband recently dead of a heart attack. For the sake of understanding, we felt it critical to search for examples in which the contributions of each sort of process could be distinguished (Kleinman, Eisenberg, and Good, 1978).

As well, there were questions of practical import. We wondered to what extent the misidentification or lack of identification of couvade could lead to prolonged patient morbidity, to iatrogenic morbidity, or to increased cost to the patient or to the health care system. We wondered about the extent to which the phenomenon would be recognized or not and to what extent recognition would lead to behavior designed to be helpful. If the phenomenon was not recognized, we wanted to know why. Was this due to lack of a construct or a diagnostic category, failure to obtain appropriate data to fill the category, or what?

The couvade condition presents a potent model for eleven reasons:

1. It is clearly psychosociogenic (the husband is not pregnant, and the symptoms arise in the setting of someone else's biological change, the expectant woman's).

2. It is so in a way in which the symptoms clearly relate to the psychosocial process involved, pregnancy in the family.

3. The phenomena involved are discrete and self-limited.

4. The phenomena involved are amenable to study through the use of records.

5. It is common.

6. It relates to a normal life cycle event.

7. It has fascinating psychodynamic implications.

8. It relates to symptomatology that habitually is treated by adult physicians in routine fashion.

9. Its detection rests on the detection of key data, such as the pregnancy of the mate.

10. Treatment of the symptoms usually involves further evaluation and/or concrete action such as prescribing antacids, doing

minor surgery, or the like. Thus the related behaviors are readily detectable.

11. It is easy to identify persons at risk.

We will now briefly tell you something about couvade and its history, review some of the prior clinical studies and some of the problems with them, and then review our design and results.

HISTORY OF COUVADE STUDIES

The term "couvade" comes from the French (Basque) *couver*, meaning "brood" or "hatch." It refers to symptoms, signs, or rituals in which men undergo experiences analogous to and resembling those that women experience during pregnancy or later.

Plutarch provided an early description of couvade, and it was described by Diodorus Siculus in 60 B.C. in Corsica. Since that time it has been found in dozens of separate cultures. Munroe, Munroe, and Whiting (1973) cite Marco Polo's writing concerning Chinese Turkistan:

> And in this province the custom is that when ladies have been confined giving birth to a child, they wash him and wrap him up in clothes and the Lord of the Lady gets into the bed, keeps the infant that is born with him and lies in the bed forty days without getting up from the bed except for important necessary duties . . . and his wife, as soon as she has given birth to her child, she gets up from the bed as soon as she can and does all the duty of the house and waits on her Lord, taking him food and drink, the time he is in the bed, as if he himself had born the child.

Trethowan (1972) cites references to couvade symptoms by Francis Bacon, by James Primrose, and by several restoration playwrights. He quotes Wilkins in *The Miserys of Enforced Marriage* in 1607, "I have got thee with child in my conscience and, like a kind husband, methinks I breeded for thee. For I am already sick at my stomach and long extremely."

Trethowan (1972) quotes Robert Heath in 1650:

> We observe each living husband, when the wife
> Is laboring by a strange reciproque strife

Doth sympathizing sicken; and 't maybe
In law they are one in divinity.

BRIEF REVIEW OF COUVADE STUDIES

Sir Edward Tylor (1865) described the ritual and named it couvade. Subsequently each generation of anthropologists has dealt with it using the prevailing explanatory mode of the day. Thus Frazer (1910) focused on the relationship between father and child and the role of sympathetic magic; Dawson (1929) used it as evidence of cultural diffusion. Malinowski (1927) suggested that it was a functional device of biological value in representing the role of the individual and the family. Psychologists including Freud, Reik (1931), and Bettelheim (1962) have presented views based on psychodynamic interpretations such as that these phenomena represent parturition envy, latent homosexuality, identification with women with resultant ambivalence and hostility, and conversion of such conflicts and ambivalences. These are not exclusive or exhaustive explanations (see also Munroe, Munroe, and Nerlove, 1973; Munroe, Munroe, and Whiting, 1973; and Evans, 1951).

The most influential modern writers on this subject are Trethowan and the Munroes. Trethowan's most central role has been clinical and scholarly, in providing case studies, early incidence data and history (see Enoch, Trethowan, and Barker, 1967; Trethowan, 1968). Secondarily he has summarized views on his own clinical psychiatric approach. In brief, he argues that three explanations have merit: (1) ambivalence in relation to the pregnancy with repressed hostility, (2) identification with the pregnant woman, (3) and parturition envy. Interestingly, Trethowan states that the importance of the couvade syndrome is in what it teaches about psychodynamics:

> . . . [concerning its] importance, this is not the outcome of its being even relatively rarely a severe source of discomfort or because it occasionally leads to diagnostic confusion. Rather it is important in that it occurs at all and in its occurrence, helps to throw some light upon the dynamics of family relationships. (Trethowan, 1972, p. 91)

In so arguing, he lacks the central data that might permit an assessment of import on solid scientific grounds — incidence data drawn from a population-based sample; a broad survey that reflects the variety of the presentations; a method that shows both the direct effects, in morbidity, and the indirect effects due to the costs, undue testing, and side effects of mislabeling. This sort of omission is the rule in studies of syndromes done by academicians in hospital centers. Only data derived from typical populations with defined populations at risk, which permit examination of the whole of the care process rather than of the isolated bit performed by the academic in question, can correct this sort of "numerator only" fallacy.

The contributions of the Munroes are worthy of mention (and not only for their elegance). In brief, they show that a specific psychological hypothesis can be meaningfully explored through combined use of cross-cultural survey and intensive psychological study of sample cultures. In their view, the prevalence of couvade ritual is most likely to be high in those cultures in which the infant is closely associated with the mother in the stages of development of the self-image but later is torn from the mother and put into a hypermasculine role. They looked for cultures with these characteristics, and in several they tested specifically for cross-sex identity, confirming their hypothesis (Munroe and Munroe, 1971).

Lipkin's view is that the necessary data to resolve the question of the psychological mechanisms are not yet available and further study is warranted. Lipkin leans to a view that combines depth psychological and structuralist notions. He suspects that the couvade phenomenon represents social triggering of a psychological mechanism in certain vulnerable men. These are men who, by virtue of their cultural background and their personal development and biology, experience some aspects of their symbolic and affective selves through sensation rather than through conscious awareness of feeling. They then engage in complex relationships to this perception and involve others such as health care personnel in ways both culturally and idiosyncratically determined. In this, the most significant activities are the covert or metacommunications between provider and patient, the one using body language of somaticization, the other using illness and healing languages — medicalization — to communicate and interact. Such complex communications are universal and necessary. They cannot necessarily be translated into direct talk by the participants. Thus, the actions of each are necessary and must be understood both for what they represent and for what they are.

In parallel with these theoretical views, a series of clinical studies documented couvade symptoms in expectant fathers in England and the United States.

Freeman (1951) studied six cases in which pregnancy was a precipitant of mental illness and noted that two of the men suffered with somatic complaints.

Curtis (1955) followed up on World War II findings that expectant fatherhood, in the military, was related to frequent "psychosomatic" problems and found that 22 of 55 men developed gastrointestinal symptoms of anorexia, nausea, epigastric pain, diarrhea, constipation, headaches, and dizziness. This study was uncontrolled, and the nature of the population was poorly defined.

Trethowan and Conlon (1965) conducted the first large study that attempted some control. Three hundred and twenty-seven fathers whose wives had just been delivered of infants were compared with 321 married men matched for social and occupational class and age range. They were given a symptom checklist and questions about the nature of the symptoms. Compared with the controls, a large number of expectant fathers suffered from indigestion, nausea, appetite change, diarrhea, constipation, toothache, and/or backache. As well there was an increase in depression, tension, insomnia, and irritability. They found an overall frequency of 11 percent of expectant fathers who may have had some psychogenic symptoms. This study failed to exclude concomitant disease that might otherwise account for the symptoms. A second limitation was the retrospective self-report method of the questionnaire that would tend to lead to underreporting.

Liebenberg (1973) studied a group of husbands who had similar symptoms. She estimated a 65 percent frequency but had no controls and stated no symptom criteria. A number of other studies, each of which was poorly controlled, found the phenomena in the 10 to 60 percent range (Dickens and Trethowan, 1971; Munroe, Munroe, and Nerlove, 1973; Munroe, Munroe, and Whiting, 1973; Roehner, 1976).

The Munroes and co-workers (1973) reported the results of an unpublished doctoral thesis by R. L. Munroe done in the early 1960s in which 200 women in their last trimester were asked about their husband's health. Forty-one percent reported that their husbands had symptoms not present prior to the onset of pregnancy.

Davis (1977) examined 91 expectant fathers using a biased selection process and a symptom checklist. She showed that somatic symptoms correlated with race, social class, planned pregnancy, and with anxiety, which Trethowan also had noted.

Cavenar and Weddington (1978), citing two cases, argued that couvade is evidence of psychosis and an indication for hospitalization. Their paper represents an example of the prevalent tendency to generalize from the extreme cases found in the experience of specialists to the general world of medical experience in which the common entity bears little or no resemblance to the severe rare ones selected for study. Only the sort of study that is based on a defined population and sensitive enough to pick up the large majority of cases can be the basis for discussion of issues such as whether a specific symptom or perception is abnormal or defines psychosis or craziness. The definition of what is normal must derive from studies of populations as well as of individuals. Specifically the craziness of experiencing affects or conflicts as symptoms must be so examined and not only in extreme cases, such as in Cavenar's two cases. But, as we will see below, their findings are not the usual case. The "medicalization" implicit in Cavenar's paper reflects results from narrow select sampling. This is a prevalent bias in medical writing that leads to inappropriate overconcern about normal phenomena.

Thus, up to the present, many authors have found an increase in symptoms suggestive of pregnancy in varied populations of men whose wives were known to be pregnant. No study controlled for concomitant disease that could otherwise explain the symptoms. None combined a broad-based, ambulatory population with clear definition of symptoms. With these considerations in mind, we decided to do a pilot study to see if there really is such a phenomenon. As well, we hoped to get some preliminary understanding of its nature and extent and some early data to point us in directions to examine its etiology in whatever framework seemed reasonable. Our first concern was to control for the common omission of the prior studies (i.e., the possible existence of concomitant disease). Second, we decided to use a practice that was typical of the working population of a large city with respect to all classes of illness phenomena. We hoped to estimate the potential impact of these phenomena on the health care system. Thus, we are introducing the use of a tracer condition as an analytical tool for the study of psychosomatic phenomena.

DESCRIPTION OF OUR PILOT STUDY

We obtained the complete obstetrical lists for the prepaid group practice at the Joseph C. Wilson Health Center, a federally qualified Health Maintenance Organization (HMO) with population typical for the area. A systematic sample of 300 women was drawn from the 753 deliveries occurring during a 14-month period. From these 300 women, 33 couples failed to meet entrance criteria and were excluded because (1) 9 couples were unmarried; (2) 9 couples were divorced or separated at the time of delivery; (3) 5 couples had not become parents and were included incorrectly on the obstetrical lists; (4) 1 couple had had a child one year prior to the stated date; (5) 2 couples had miscarriages; and (6) 7 couples' records could not be found. We then examined the women's records and reviewed the father's records. We looked at all visits from the date of knowledge of the pregnancy to delivery.

For control, we compared these visits to two control periods for each patient. The first was the six months prior to pregnancy. The second control period was from two weeks postpartum to six months after delivery. So each case was its own control. Using the data available in the chart, we ascertained whether the symptoms and signs reported were associated with a concomitant disease as documented by some additional objective method such as laboratory evaluation.

A rating system to identify couvade condition was devised. It was defined as seeking care during the pregnancy for one or more of the symptoms listed below. We included, as couvade symptoms, those found by previous authors to be of significance. These were nausea, vomiting, loss of appetite, diarrhea, constipation, sties, abdominal pain, skin conditions, faintness, lassitude, and leg cramps. This definition of couvade symptoms is conservative, as will be seen. This is because many other sorts of symptoms that make sense were found also to fit the pattern (e.g., low back pain, urinary burning and frequency, and rectal bleeding). We omitted these for this study because they are not usually included in prior studies and because we wished to keep the case conservative, without severely distorting our sense of the phenomenology.

A third reason conservative definition is sensible was not decisive but is interesting. We recognized that if we did include back pain, for example, we would run into the problem of ghost explanation that would convince some readers that rather than experiencing what we are suggesting, a psychosociogenic symptom complex, the patients are experiencing a ghost disease. A ghost disease is a disease for which there are no direct confirmatory tests so that the practitioner can diagnose them on the basis of history alone. Such entities exist in each category of disease. Common ones include lumbosacral strain for low back pain, peptic ulcer syndrome for abdominal pain, coronary spasm for chest pain, atypical migraine for headache, and so forth. The existence of such entities permits the practitioner to deny the possibility of psychogenic origins of specific symptoms, to give the patient some discrete (face saving) explanation, some treatment, and some protection against fear of the unknown or uncertain. These explanations are sometimes, also, valid. When not, they are hard ghosts to exorcise. This is an example of inappropriate labeling not of medicalization.

Each pregnancy event was characterized independently by the authors as to the presence or absence of couvade symptoms.

OVERVIEW OF QUANTITATIVE RESULTS
OF THE PILOT STUDY

Data were analyzed using one-way and multivariate analysis of variance. Interrater reliability was 92 percent for couvade symptoms. The men identified as having couvade were those seeking care for one or more couvade symptoms. The mean age of our samples was 28.7 (range 19 to 49) years of age. Hollingshead Education Class was 3 (range 1 to 7; class 3 is partial college education), Occupation was 4 (range 1 to 7; class 4 is clerical, sales workers, technicians), and Social Position was 3 (range 1 to 5); thus these were typical urban men. These men had an average of 2.5 prior children (range 0 to 7) and had attended childbirth education classes in one-half of the cases.

Sixty of our 267 men had couvade symptoms for which they sought care. This is 22.5 percent, or a prevalence of 225 per 1,000 (of men whose wives are pregnant).

Age accounted for little variance with respect to distribution of couvade symptoms, although there is a tendency for younger men to seek more assistance in dealing with couvade symptoms.

Education level was important in that men with less education (high school or less) tended to have more couvade symptoms than the more educated men. Interestingly, more educated men did have an increase of symptoms as well during pregnancy. They were far vaguer and less clearly defined complaints, such as feeling run down. We interpreted this, preliminarily, to indicate a higher degree of defendedness. Those with none or more than three children had more couvade symptoms than those with one to three children.

Attendance at childbirth education classes and existence of pregnancy complications did not account for presence or absence of couvade symptoms. This is interesting in that those who subscribed to a model of pregnancy as a general "stressor" might suppose that those with pregnancy complications in their mate might be more, or less, likely to develop symptoms. This was not the case. Similarly, it might be hypothesized that childbirth education classes would be evidence of greater or lesser involvement with the pregnancy with higher or lower adaptiveness. These preliminary data do not support any such hypotheses. However, the numbers are small.

Turning to *care seeking behavior* we found that those with no couvade symptoms maintained a relatively constant level of visits before, during, and after the pregnancy of their wives. In contrast, those with couvade symptoms had a highly significant twofold increase in visits.

The number of symptoms for each time period differed significantly. The men with couvade symptoms had more symptoms to begin with, and during pregnancy they reported four times as many symptoms. This difference was highly significant. Thus, there was clearly a difference in illness behavior and in care seeking behavior

Mean Number of Patient-initiated Visits
by Each Time Period

	Before Pregnancy	During Pregnancy	After Pregnancy
No Couvade	0.70	0.69	0.79
Couvade	1.00	2.15	0.77

Before pregnancy = 6 months prior to onset of pregnancy; After pregnancy = 2 weeks to 6 months after delivery; couvade vs. no couvade difference significant at 0.001 level during pregnancy.

between the groups. The finding that men with couvade had more symptoms to begin with is not surprising if couvade is viewed as a coping method triggered now in a specific and analyzable setting. Men who tend to use the care system in coping might be expected to continue to do so. Men who experience themselves through symptoms might be expected to continue to do so.

The finding that the increase in symptoms was fourfold is reassuring in that it supports the fact that something is really happening. That there was some increase is tautologic in that this group is selected for having symptoms for which they seek care. The objection that this all might simply be an arbitrary selection of those with more symptoms does not hold for these reasons: because the increase is so high, because the symptoms have meaning, and because the cases are their own controls. Nevertheless, we are doing a second study with a variety of additional controls.

The character of response by the medical personnel also was examined. One hundred and seventy-nine of the 267 expectant fathers visited the health center during the pregnancy period. In 85.5 percent of these cases, no note was made of the expectant fatherhood of the patient.

Of the men with couvade symptoms, 21.7 percent were recognized as expectant fathers. Analysis was done to see if the increased frequency of recognition of expectant fatherhood was due to the greater number of visits by those with couvade symptoms. This turned out to be the case. When adjustment for number of visits was made, the difference of recording of recognition that the man's mate was pregnant between the two groups no longer was significant. What this shows is that the physicians did not record the fact of the wife's pregnancy. We do not know to what extent they knew of it but did not choose to put it down in the chart. To the extent they were unaware of the wife's pregnancy, they could not be expected to connect it with the man's symptoms.

Physicians prescribed medication for those with couvade symptoms twice as often as for those without. This is elaborated below.

However, there were no significant differences between those with couvade and those without couvade with respect to the frequency of reassurance, of counseling, of referral, or of notation of symptoms of anxiety, tension, or irritability. None of these men was noted to be referred to a mental health worker or psychiatrist. Although it is often noted that men may become psychotic during pregnancy of their wives (Towne and Afterman, 1955; Freeman, 1951; Wainwright, 1966), this did not happen in this sample of 267. It was unseen in this population.

OVERVIEW OF QUALITATIVE RESULTS OF OUR STUDY

We wish now to give you some feeling for the nature of our qualitative findings concerning care giving behavior and concerning some of the cases.

First, what were the prescriptions given? Case by case analysis was undertaken by Lipkin to ascertain what medications were prescribed and which seemed of dubious indication based on the clinical data. In the 60 cases, the following items were prescribed without clear medical indication in the chart, if one accepts the identification of the patient's condition as couvade rather than the unproved diagnosis given: Periactin, sitzbaths, milk of magnesia, indomethacin (a potent anti-inflammatory drug with potentially lethal side effects), tetracycline, Empirin with codeine (a narcotic), cortisone, erythromycin, Librax, Tylenol with codeine, Donnatol, Valium, hydrocortisone, Sudafed, Lomotil, Antivert, salicylic acid soaks, Mylanta, Donnagel, and epinephrine. Of these, most are minor, a few have significant side effects in the exceptional case, and a few — indomethacin, codeine, cortisone, prednisone, and epinephrine — are potent and potentially seriously harmful medications. The tests done included 14 chest radiographs, 18 complete blood cell counts, five sigmoidoscopies, a gallbladder series, an upper gastrointestinal series, and comparable numbers of electrocardiograms, urinalyses, differential blood cell counts, stool guaiacs, lipid screens, and glucose tests, among others. Some of these were unnecessary. As such, they represent a significant cost that is partially avoidable. Minor surgery was done in five men for removal of long present, harmless cysts.

Symptoms for which care was sought were counted as couvade only if they fitted the narrow criteria derived from the literature and described above. However, a number of men had other symptoms of ankle swelling and water retention (in which these are *not* noted as present on physical examination), back pain, retrosternal burning, genital burning and itching, urinary burning, groin pain, knee pain and upper leg pain, blood in the saliva, and dizziness when laughing. One patient reported abdominal pain, cysts, and knee swelling. He had the cysts removed and had no complaints on his next visit. Several patients with abdominal cramping reported rectal bleeding that was never confirmed despite adequate testing.

Some of the constellations of symptoms and historical data were fascinating. One patient reported chest pain as if "something was pushing out." He also had urinary burning and abdominal pain. His abdominal pain seemed to be "sinking into his bladder." One patient had chest pain, warts, moles (i.e., growths), constipation/diarrhea, bright red blood in his stool, and negative results on physical evaluation.

A final, fascinating patient reported "upper leg pain." It was noted elsewhere in his chart that he had suffered from congenital displacement of his hips. As an infant, he had both legs put in a cast, which may cause pain in the infants so treated.

An informal check on symptoms that patients felt but did not seek care for was done. Lipkin questioned five members of the sample who were his patients and who were in the no-couvade category. During visits for other reasons, he asked about the presence of any unusual symptoms during their wives' pregnancy. Two of the five (doctors) said that they had had symptoms that had been self-limited. They had not attempted to seek care because they knew routine complaints required a one-month wait for an appointment. Clearly, our numbers underestimate the frequency of symptoms. They are, however, reasonable reflections of the combination of care obtaining behavior of our patients and the recording behaviors of our doctors.

Discussion of such events with patients, with students, and with colleagues, and even with psychiatrists, characteristically produces one of several reactions. A frequent reaction is laughter. Another is disinterest or denial. Psychiatrists rarely encounter these patients in their work (e.g., the referral rate for these patients was lower than for the nonpatients). None of these 60 men saw a psychiatrist or mental health worker for or with their complaints. Thus mental health workers could not recognize their prevalence. When they do see them, there is an ecologic fallacious relation to the craziness that led the patient to the psychiatrist. That is, it is not the couvade, but the craziness, that send them to the psychiatrist. The psychiatrist, who sees people with craziness every day, but rarely encounters couvade, connects the two as occurring together.

A critical lesson of our data is that this is a problem that is clearly not in the domain of the mental health specialist. None of the 60 men with couvade had contact with a mental health specialist. Only primary care physicians see these sorts of problems in their common forms. Specialists see them in extreme forms. Only primary care personnel can intervene in the least costly ways, and only those who study these phenomena in general settings among the population at large can comment on what is normal about them and what is pathological or prognostic of further difficulty. Examination of the extreme forms may illuminate facets of the processes involved but may equally overshadow them or introduce false connections. This sampling error is often confused with medicalization.

In Lipkin's personal practice experience with patients with this phenomenon, even those who are in psychotherapy rarely connect the nature of their symptoms with their wives' pregnancy. This suggests that active denial is playing a role and that conversion may be a factor in some cases. The patient whose upper leg pain may be reminiscent of his infantile neonatal pains illustrates this. During his wife's pregnancy, a second patient developed a pregnancylike posture in which his abdomen was protuberant and his hips rotated forward. He complained of back pain. Attempts to alter his posture through exercise and direct postural awareness were unsuccessful. Discussion of his role in the pregnancy, without any suggestion of a relationship to his illness, resulted in a change in posture and elimination of pain over the next two days.

CONCLUSIONS AND COMMENTS

We found a prevalence of 225/1,000 for couvade symptomatology in a population of expectant fathers. These are men without concomitant disease to explain the symptoms. The number of symptoms is increased in these men. The number of their visits to health care personnel is increased. They are given more treatments than controls. Many of the tests and procedures done for them were unnecessary and costly. There was correlation with lack of education, with being a younger father, and with having either no children or a considerable number of children and the development of these symptoms.

We intentionally used conservative criteria for the couvade syndrome to convince ourselves that the phenomenon exists. This may lead to an underestimate of the prevalence. Cases occurred in which no alternative diagnosis was made, symptoms were increased, and the symptoms described were suggestive of pregnancy-like events but experienced farther away in the body than the usual abdominal couvade. Examples included the patient mentioned above with chest pain that felt "like something is pushing out"; several patients who reported bright red blood in their stool in whom no trace of blood was found in the stool, rectum, or colon; and a patient who reported a stuffed head "as if something is filling it up and pushing down."

Lipkin views such symptoms in two basic ways. First they are felt. Second they can be body language. Why such language arises, what the *emic* and what the *etic* (based on the distinction of phonemic and phonetic or universal and local) (Serpell, 1982) elements are, and how they complexly reflect biology, personality, and culture are beyond the scope of this chapter. But such questions fascinate us.

With respect to medicalization, the lesson of such events is obvious. The problem is one of too *narrow* a taxonomy. Janzen argues this by comparing Bantu and other medical systems that bridge the physical and moral. Our case derives from the clinical facts. We here document an omission, typical of a class of omissions, and suggest that the price of such omission may be great.

This raises the following issues. First, what is the historical basis of such omission and narrowing? What elements are political; what are scientific? Have the politics distorted the science? Or vice versa! Second, are there other sorts of reasons for such omissions, such as human ecologic limitations or difficulties in dealing with over-complex explanatory or action modes? Other theoretic questions also arise in this context. Foremost of these is the relation of such illness episodes and biological and psychological explanatory modes. Such issues are discussed in Chapter 9.

Our use of chart review is biased by the incompleteness of recording. Many of the charts suggested spotty recording of symptoms. As well, this method detects only those who obtained care. We missed those who were sick but either did not seek medical care, sought care outside our system, or failed to obtain sought care. Finally, we did not directly observe patients and personnel. Hence all conclusions must be tentative concerning the actual interactions. But the trend of these omissions is to *under*estimate frequencies.

Providers seemed to react to the symptoms in predictable disease-related ways. Thus, those presenting with abdominal pain or cramping were dealt with as if they had one or several disorders from the list of differential diagnostic physical disorders that present as abdominal pain (not including couvade), such as peptic ulcer syndrome. They were given tests relevant to these differential diagnostic items, which seems reasonable and appropriate. Then, despite the absence of positive findings, many of them were treated according to some presumed diagnosis or given a ghost diagnosis. They were given medications, generally mild, although not in every case harmless, ones. They were also subjected to procedures, generally, but not always, safe ones. Some were, however, not pleasant. In a few cases the procedures or prescriptions were potentially harmful. In most cases, providers failed to record relevant data concerning the life context of the patient and relevant supporting data concerning their developmental histories. This made it improbable that the providers would make an appropriate assessment. To what extent this is due to their ignorance of this diagnostic possibility was not determined. A prospective study that includes direct observation of actual provider findings as opposed to information in the charts and that assesses personnel attitudes and knowledge of couvade seems indicated.

With respect to the themes of this book, we have illustrated a situation in which the biotechnical orientation of care providers in a typical large practice has resulted in the failure to identify an illness resulting from a change in life cycle and context. The costs of this include increased frequency of visits by these patients, increased prescription of medication (some of it hazardous), and the cost and discomfort of unneeded tests. Failure to recognize the causes of the visits may result in decreased opportunity to help on the part of the provider, although this point is moot since we are not sure what helps or if help is needed even though it is sought. We have suggested this relates complexly to medicalization in the sense that medical interest must at least extend to this normal life cycle event, and by extrapolation, to others. We show here that the issue is one of appropriate labeling and models and data identification and that denial of the relations of psychological, biological, and social events can only add to iatrogenic harm rather than eliminate it. In this respect, the views of Illich (1976), Carlson (1975), Szasz (1961), and the like, while well intended, are inadequate.

Because they are merely reactive to a *too narrow* system, their reactions also are too narrow.

Extrapolated across the national birth rate, the financial costs of this example can be estimated to be enormous. According to World Population Estimates, 1979, published by the Environmental Fund, the national birth rate is 14.8/1,000. If the population is 200 million, that is about 3 million births per year. If couvade phenomena drive 20 percent of men to seek care, that is about one-half million such cases per year. If these each have three visits, that is over a million visits per year. If they have twice the normal amount of medicine prescribed, consider the probable costs (even if each prescription costs a low $2.00). Consider the attendant tests. Consider the side effects of the medications. Most, even mild, medications have serious side effects at a rate of one event per thousand or two thousand. So across the nation, serious side effects are highly likely to occur. Consider finally that even if our estimates are off by an order of magnitude (remembering that our feeling is that our estimates are low, that we did not detect those who self-medicated), the magnitude of the costs and risks still remains large.

As well, this is just one small example of this sort of phenomenon. Lipkin, Markovics, and Dohring (1977) showed that patients with overt, complex psychosomatic symptoms constituted about 4 percent of a large HMO practice. There is an unexplored universe of such phenomena waiting to be described.

We think it fair to conclude that a disease orientation per se unless it includes culturally and personally (psychogenically) determined diseases (i.e., illnesses) can be significantly wasteful, may fail to provide appropriate help, and will at varied but real rates be productive of iatrogenic problems and needless cost.

REFERENCES

Bettelheim, B. 1962. *Symbolic Wounds: Puberty Rites and the Envious Male.* New York: Colliers.

Carlson, R. 1975. *The End of Medicine.* New York: Wiley-Interscience.

Cavenar, J. O., Jr., and Weddington, W. W., Jr. 1978. Abdominal Pain in Expectant Fathers. *Psychomatics* 19:761-68.

Curtis, J. 1955. A Psychiatric Study of 55 Expectant Fathers. *U.S. Armed Forces Med. J.* 6:937-50.

Davis, O. 1977. Moods and Symptoms of Expectant Fathers during the Course of Pregnancy: A Study of the Crisis Perspective of Expectant Fatherhood.

Ph.D. dissertation, University of North Carolina at Greensboro.

Dawson, W. R. 1929. *The Custom of Couvade*. Manchester: Manchester University Press.

Dickens, G., and Trethowan, W. H. 1971. Cravings and Aversions during Pregnancy. *J. Psychosom. Res.* 15:259-68.

Enoch, M.; Trethowan, W.; and Barker, J. 1967. The Couvade Syndrome. In *Some Uncommon Psychiatric Symptoms*, ed. M. O. Enoch and W. M. Trethowan. Baltimore: Williams & Wilkins.

Evans, W. N. 1951. Simulated Pregnancy in a Male. *Psychoanalytic Quarterly* 20:165-78.

Feinstein, A. 1967. *Clinical Judgment*. Baltimore: Williams & Wilkins.

Frazer, J. G. 1910. *Totemism and Exogamy*, Vol. 4. London: Macmillan.

Freeman, T. 1951. Pregnancy as a Precipitant of Mental Illness in Men. *Brit. J. Med. Psych.* 24:49-54.

Freud, S. *Standard Edition*, Vols. 2 and 9, ed. E. Jones. London: Institute of Psychoanalysis.

Hoeper, E. 1979. Observations on the Impact of Psychiatric Disorder upon Primary Medical Care. In *Mental Health Services in General Health Care*. Washington, D.C.: National Academy of Sciences.

Illich, I. 1976. *Medical Nemesis: The Expropriation of Health*. New York: Pantheon.

Kleinman, A.; Eisenberg, L.; Good, B. 1978. Culture, Illness and Care. *Ann. Intern. Med.* 88:251-58.

Knowles, J. 1977. *Doing Better and Feeling Worse*. New York: Norton.

Liebenberg, B. 1973. Expectant Fathers. In *Psychological Aspects of a First Pregnancy and Early Post Natal Adaptation*, ed. P. Shereshefsky and L. Yarrlo. New York: Raven Press.

Lipkin, M., Jr., and Kupka, K. 1982. *Psychosocial Factors Affecting Health*. New York: Praeger.

Lipkin, M., Jr., and Lamb, G. S. 1982. The Couvade Syndrome: An Epidemiological Study. *Ann. Intern. Med.* 96(61).

Lipkin, M., Jr.; Markovics, C.; and Dohring, D. 1977. *Integrating Mental Health Services in an HMO: Implementing a Holistic Approach*. Group Health Institute.

Malinowski, B. 1927. *Sex and Repression in Savage Society*. New York: Harcourt, Brace.

Mechanic, D. 1961. The Concept of Illness Behavior. *J. Chronic Dis.* 15:189-94.

Munroe, R. L., and Munroe, R. H. 1971. Male Pregnancy Symptoms and Cross Sex Identity in Three Societies. *J. Soc. Psychol.* 84:11-25.

Munroe, R. L.; Munroe, R. H.; and Nerlove, S. B. 1973. Male Pregnancy Symptoms and Cross Sex Identity: Two Replications. *J. Soc. Psychol.* 89:147-48.

Munroe, R. L.; Munroe, R. H.; and Whiting, J. W. M. 1973. The Couvade: A Psychological Analysis. *Ethos* 1(1):30-74.

Parsons, T. 1951. *The Social System*. Glencoe, Ill.: Free Press.

Regier, D. 1979. Nature and Scope of Mental Health Problems in Primary Care. In *Mental Health Services in General Health Care*, Washington, D.C.: National Academy of Sciences.

Reik, T. 1931. *Ritual.* New York: Norton.

Roehner, J. 1976. Fatherhood in Pregnancy and Birth. *J. Nurse-Midwifery* 21:13-18.

Schlesinger, H.; Mumford, E.; and Glass, G. 1979. Problems in Analyzing the Cost-Offset in Providing Mental Health Services in Primary Care Settings. In *Mental Health Services in General Health Care*. Washington, D.C.: National Academy of Sciences.

Serpell, R. 1982. Psychosocial Constructs, Health Records and the Sociocultural Environment. In *Psychosocial Problems Affecting Health*, ed. M. Lipkin, Jr., and K. Kupka. New York: Praeger.

Shepherd, M. 1979. Mental Health as an Integrant of Primary Care. In *Mental Health Services in General Health Care*, Vol. 1. Washington, D.C.: National Academy of Sciences.

Szasz, T. 1961. *Myth of Mental Illness.* New York: Delta.

Towne, R. D., and Afterman, J. 1955. Psychosis in Males Related to Parenthood. *Bull. Menninger Clin.* 19:19-26.

Trethowan, W. H. 1968. The Couvade Syndrome – Some Further Observations. *J. Psychosom. Res.* 12:107-15.

Trethowan, W. H. 1972. The Couvade Syndrome. In *Modern Perspectives in Psycho-Obstetrics*, ed. J. Howells. New York: Brunner/Mazel.

Trethowan, W. H., and Conlon, M. F. 1965. The Couvade Syndrome. *Brit. J. Psychiatry* 3:57-66.

Tylor, E. B. 1865. *Researches into the Early History of Mankind and the Development of Civilization*, 2nd ed. London: Murray.

Wainwright, W. H. 1966. Fatherhood as a Precipitant of Mental Illness. *Am. J. Psychiatry* 123:40-44.

Wersinger, R. D., and Roberts, J. S. 1977. Comparative Analyses of the Enrollments and Utilization Experience of a Federally Qualified Prepaid HMO: the First Three Years' Experience. *Proceedings 27th Annual Group Health Institute*, pp. 232-48.

7

ON CHANGES IN WEIGHT
OF EXPECTANT FATHERS

Ayala Gabriel

The birth of a first child is a transition, for both women *and* men, from one social status to another, that is, from childless individuals to that of parents. From the moment that the pregnancy is confirmed, husbands and wives seek and receive recognition and support for their status as expectant parents. Throughout the pregnancy both husbands and wives participate in a variety of social, familial, medical, and paramedical activities in which they seek and receive support for their status.

Change of weight is one of the ways that men may use in social interaction to present themselves as expectant fathers and be acknowledged in this status. During a study of the transition to parenthood among 53 white, middle-class couples in Rochester, New York, I observed the concern of men with weight changes. The aim of the study was to consider the birth of the first child as a focal event for couples' allocations and adjustments of occupational and domestic roles. Each husband and wife were interviewed together twice before and twice after the birth, at the couple's house. The topic of change of weight was frequently brought up by husbands

This paper forms part of the author's Ph.D. dissertation work at the University of Rochester (Gabriel, 1980). This research was supported by NIMH Research Fellowship Award 5 F31 MH07468-02 MP.

in the prenatal interviews, and I thought that it might be indicative of a general phenomenon. But because the topic came up incidentally, my observations about it should be regarded as suggestive rather than conclusive.

The transition to parenthood is marked by three major changes: (1) physiological, (2) psychological, and (3) social. Women experience all three changes, but men experience only the last two. Women's physiological change ensures them social recognition of their status and continued support for it from the moment that the pregnancy becomes noticeable. As Rubin describes it, "once the pregnancy becomes more apparent the behavior of others toward her confirm the fact that she is pregnant" (1969, p. 328). For men, the transition to parenthood is a different experience. Medical confirmation of the pregnancy puts the husband in the liminal stage; he becomes an expectant father. *He* knows it, but others do not, unless he tells them. Some husbands are aware of this difference. As one husband said: "Everyone can see that *she* is expecting a baby." But, if he wanted people to know, he had to tell them.

Men in my study wanted others to know that they were expectant fathers. I suggest that gain and loss of weight are expressions of a wish to be recognized in the status of expectant fathers. Others will notice this change in the husbands just as they will notice the women's pregnancies. Whereas the women's physical change will be noticed directly, the men's change of weight allows them to announce their new status as expectant fathers. When they are asked about their gain or loss of weight, they are likely to use it to introduce the subject of the pregnancy. Even if they are not asked, they may use the weight phenomenon to lead up to a mention of their expectant fatherhood. In a social encounter they would typically say, "I had to lose weight, because I have to be in good shape so that when the kid is born I can go out and play with him."

Women act in an entirely analogous way when they wear maternity clothes long before bodily changes are apparent. That, too, announces the new status of expectant mother.

In my study I encountered both men who gained weight and men who lost weight. I came across more cases of loss of weight and intentions to lose weight. The reasons that men gave for loss of weight were mostly related to responsibilities in their coming parental status, but some also referred directly to the pregnancy.

Mostly, men said they lost weight because they were going to be fathers and had to be in good health and "shape."

The following examples will illustrate these concerns. An expectant father told me in our second prenatal interview that he went to see his physician to have a total physical examination and to consult with him on a diet since he wished to lose weight. His physician told him that he was in perfect health and did not need a diet as he was not in any way overweight. He told me that the physician asked him why he wanted to lose weight: "I told him (the physician) that I feel responsible. I want to be in good health because we are expecting a baby. All of a sudden I think about it, about my mortality." In spite of what his physician said, the man lost weight and took up jogging. After his child was born, he did not mention the need to lose weight anymore but continued the jogging.

Another man told me that he decided to lose weight because he had pains in his chest and feared some heart trouble. He decided later that the pains were due to the fact that he had moved a lot of heavy furniture, but even so he still worried about his weight. He decided that to lose weight was a good idea none the less, because he wanted his child to get a father in good health. He also mentioned that he told some of his colleagues at work both about the incident of the chest pain and about the decision to lose weight and that he said to them jokingly: "What kind of a father is this child going to have if I don't take care of myself?"

In another family the man told me that he lost weight so that he would be able to play baseball with his child. The interesting thing is that, now that his child is almost two years old, this man is back at his somewhat heavy weight and does not seem to be bothered by it when he plays with his child.

Another man in the study told the prenatal class instructor that the reason that he lost weight was very prosaic: They stopped buying food that was not nutritious so that his wife would eat only well-balanced meals. He rationalized that if he ate "junk" food his wife would be tempted to eat it as well and that would not be good for the baby. Later on, he commented that the prenatal class instructor was paying more attention to the women in the class than to the men. He liked the classes, he said, but felt that they did not provide sufficient opportunities for men to express themselves. He said: "They (the class instructors) put the women on the pedestal and forget all about the men."

One expectant father lost a lot of weight between the first and second prenatal interviews. I commented on his changed appearance, and he said: "Isn't that funny? Joyce is pregnant and I am losing all this weight." One of the men who lost weight said very clearly and explicitly that he wanted others to know that he is an expectant father: "I want everyone to know that we are going to have a baby. I know that work is work, but I want them [my colleagues] all to know."

Men who gained weight during their wife's pregnancy related it to pregnancy diet prescriptions and proscriptions, that is, they now ate only well-balanced meals and cut out food that was regarded as harmful. One man who gained a lot of weight during his wife's pregnancy said: "I joke about it. I tell the guys that I do all the cooking now. I have to make sure that she gets well-balanced meals." Another man said that when people commented on his changed appearance, he said: "Well it is a fact: my wife is pregnant and I gain all this weight." He and his wife joked about it, and his wife said: "After the baby is born we are both going on a diet."

Evidently, men found occasion to discuss pregnancy in the context of both weight loss and weight gain. This suggests that what mattered was the opportunity weight change gave them for announcing and reannouncing their coming parental status. This seemed more important than the explicit purpose the men gave for the change.

Another indication of this function of weight change is that men seemed to lose interest in the subject after the birth of the child. During the pregnancy men seemed much more concerned with weight than women. They frequently discussed both their own and their wives' weight, whereas women seemed rather matter-of-fact about it. After the birth of the child the concern with weight loss shifted to the women, who became concerned with their appearances. If the only motivation for weight change had been the health reasons stated explicitly, one would have expected men's interest in weight loss to continue after the baby was born.

A latent motivation of change in weight apparently is to receive social recognition and support as expectant fathers. Men may want this acknowledgement by others because it is difficult to accomplish the transition to parenthood alone (Kimball, 1975). They know themselves to be expectant fathers, but they also want "to be known" as such (Fortes, 1973).

If change of weight during their wives' pregnancy is an expression of male envy, I believe that it is more envy of social recognition than envy of the actual biological process (Bettelheim, 1962). Evidence for this is that among the men who wished to lose weight only a few said that they wished that they could be pregnant; more men said that they definitely would not have liked to be pregnant and were glad that they were spared from what seemed to them a physical ordeal.

For the men in my study, change of weight appeared to serve a function similar to that of ritual in small-scale societies, that is, it marked their passage from the status of childless individuals to the status of fathers.

Men's change of weight might be regarded as part of the "rites of passage." The purpose of such rites is to "enable the individual to pass from one social status to another which is equally defined" (van Gennep, 1975, p. 3). Turner (1967) points out that rites of passage exist in all societies but may be expressed in different ways. In small-scale societies, these rites tend to be institutionalized, formal, explicit, and bound up with systems of religious beliefs. In my study, I found that some "rites of passage" that accompany transition to parenthood are ceremonial and formal, such as baby showers, but others, such as the announcement of pregnancy to the couple's parents, are not. The change of weight of expectant fathers is an instance of such an informal, noninstitutionalized "rite of passage."

REFERENCES

Bettelheim, B. 1962. *Symbolic Wounds: Puberty Rites and the Envious Male.* New York: Colliers.

Fortes, M. 1973. On the Concept of the Person among the Tallensi. In *La Notion de Personne en Afrique Noire*, ed. G. Dieterlen. Paris: Editions du Centre National de la Recherche Scientifique.

Gabriel, A. 1980. Parenthood by Choice: Transition to Parenthood among 53 White Middle-Class Couples in Rochester, New York. Ph.D. dissertation, University of Rochester.

Kimball, S. T. 1967. Introduction. In *The Rites of Passage*, ed. A. van Gennep. Chicago: University of Chicago Press.

Rubin, R. 1969. Some Aspects of Childbearing. In *Current Concepts in Clinical Nursing*, Vol. II, ed. B. S. Bergersen et al. St. Louis: Mosby.

Turner, V. 1967. *The Forest of Symbols.* Ithaca, N.Y.: Cornell University Press.

van Gennep, A. 1978. *The Rites of Passage.* Chicago: University of Chicago Press.

8

MEDICALIZATION, LABELING, AND COUVADE

Dean Harper

DEFINITION OF MEDICALIZATION

"Medicalization" is not yet found in any dictionaries, but we can predict, with some certainty, that it will be in the future. The suffix "-ize" means "to make" or "to do." The suffix "-ion" means "the act of." Thus, "medicalization" can be defined as "the act of making medical."

This definition raises three questions:

1. What is it that is made medical?
2. What does it mean to make something medical?
3. How does the process of making something medical occur?

In the first part of this chapter, I will discuss the notion of medicalization and attempt to answer these questions; then I will relate the discussion to sociological analyses of behavior, especially that of deviant behavior. Finally I will relate the discussion to couvade.

In this definition, something is left out; it should be "the act of making X medical," with the X referring to that which is made medical. At first, medicalization would seem to suggest some physical process, such as making a piece of wood into a table — which would suggest a comparable term "tablization" — the act of making a table.

THE SOCIAL NATURE OF MEDICALIZATION

It is possible that in medicalization, some physical transformation or change occurs, but more likely the transformation is social in nature. As it is used, medicalization seems to refer to a process whereby the social nature of an individual is changed or transformed *and also* the meaning or significance of some behavior (or action or phenomenon) is changed or transformed. That is to say, if Y represents the "social nature" of a person at time t_1, and if something happens to the individual, then Z represents the individual's social nature at a later time, t_2.

One example of the social nature is the set of social positions or statuses of the individual. Thus, Y consists of all of the social statuses (e.g., husband, father, store manager, member of local chamber of commerce, director on school board, president of hiking club, deacon in church), and Z consists of Y plus a new position — that of patient — that temporarily overshadows the other positions; as patient, the individual is excused from carrying out the roles of the other positions. The thing that led this individual to become a patient was a bundle of sensations and physiological events referred to as hepatitis. The initial reference to these sensations and physiological events as hepatitis was made by an individual occupying a special position that carries with it the obligation of classifying sets of symptoms and signs and assigning some label to them; in industrial countries that position and its occupant are called "physician." The symptoms and signs are labeled "hepatitis," and the individual exhibiting those symptoms and signs is now a "patient," who has the condition called "hepatitis." Whatever else has happened, medicalization (i.e., a special kind of social transformation) has occurred.

Now, for some physicians, the important and perhaps only relevant feature of this is that an expert physician has made a diagnosis and prescribed a course of treatment. In that sense, the physician is "processing" a patient and is no different from, say, an automobile mechanic diagnosing a car's problem as the need for a clutch adjustment. The mechanic keeps the car for half a day and makes the necessary repairs. In doing this, no concern is given to the car's feelings, the responses of other cars to the vicissitudes of this car, and the like, because the car, as an inanimate object, cannot participate in any of this.

But, in respect to the individual with hepatitis, sociologists and some physicians are interested in the social features of having hepatitis. Sociologists describe "having hepatitis" in terms of status movement, socialization for occupying a new status, and the like.

Still another kind of social transformation that can occur to individuals (and which might accompany the acquiring of the patient role) is a change in personality (and personality is distinct from social position). Thus, individuals, who at one time are seen and think of themselves as "healthy," now may be seen and think of themselves as "sick." Above I say "might" because such a change is not inevitable. To be seen as healthy or sick (or anything else) by others feeds and is fed by self-perception. Some individuals with a serious illness, as certified by physicians, resist the self-perception of sick and push themselves to their limits while maintaining good cheer; this may cause others to see them as "brave" and "hopeful," as not "letting their illness get them down," and so on. Others with mild or even imaginary illnesses (e.g., the "pseudocardiac patient") quickly embrace a self-view of being sick (and reinforce it by limiting their behavior and by seeking out symptoms that confirm their self-image). In turn, this can influence how others see them. Thus, a possible consequence of "having an illness" is a change in one's self-image to that of being a "sick person." This can be thought of as another instance of medicalization.

Correspondingly, as the social nature of the individual is transformed, so also is the interpretation or meaning of the events in which the individual is implicated. Thus, an individual with, say, stomach pains may try to interpret or explain those pains. It may be seen as a consequence of something that had been eaten as signifying some form of stress, or as symptomatic of some unknown disease. In the latter case, the person goes to see a doctor (unless the diagnosis of cancer is possible, in which case the individual represses the self-diagnosis in hopes that the ailment will go away). The doctor decides that the patient has a mild gastroenteritis and asserts that it will be self-limiting and self-treating; no medical treatment is required or prescribed. Thus, the individual "medicalized" his or her sensations, and the appropriateness of this was confirmed by the physician. The pains in short time do disappear; the individual did not remain in the position of patient and did not alter the self-image, but the person's physiological experience was "medicalized."

What is noted and emphasized is that whatever else it is, the process of medicalization is social. In the context of Western culture, the process can *also* be seen as an instance of scientific decision making, but here we are interested in the determinants and consequences of that decision. The decision is made in a social context and involves relations, which might be quite complex, between two or more individuals. In validating the presence of what is considered a disease, the physician is routinely doing what he or she has been trained to do and what is personally seen to be his or her task. However, the physician is doing more than this. The physician is an agent who causes the process of medicalization to occur to someone else or to something else, and thus we need to look at the relation between the medicaliz*or* and the medicaliz*ee*.

Another meaning of medicalization might be as a referent to a larger and more global process, such as might be conveyed by the expression, "the medicalization of American society." By this expression is meant the frequent occurrence of the individual events mentioned above and perhaps the inappropriate occurrence of those events. With the frequent occurrence of these events comes cultural change — a fascination with health and illness that is reflected in frequent reports in newspapers, magazines, television, and popular literature, a filtering into all aspects of life a concern with health and illness, and increased prestige for the agents of medicalization.

MEDICALIZATION: NORMATIVE OR DISRUPTIVE?

One ancillary question is: does it make sense to distinguish between correct medicalization and incorrect medicalization? In one sense this is a meaningless question. Sociologically, medicalization is a process that occurs, neither correctly nor incorrectly. However, against the standard of modern medicine, medicalization can be either correct or incorrect. This is because medicalization contains the decision by someone that the behavior or actions of someone else are pathological or physiologically based, and therefore are the subject of special concern of those in medical occupations and professions.

In attempting to detect the presence of a disease, epidemiologists talk of "false-positives" and "false-negatives." Two kinds of errors can be made: (1) deciding a disease is present when it is not (false-positive) and (2) deciding a disease is absent when it is present (false-negative). Although correct decisions can be and are made, in any particular instance the physician does not know if the decision is correct but only has some degree of confidence in the decision. The confidence may not be total or complete, even if an autopsy is performed.

In respect to medicalization, this situation can be represented in the following:

		Should the individual have been medicalized?	
		Yes	No
Has the individual been, *in fact*, medicalized?	Yes	"Correct"	"Incorrect"
	No	"Incorrect"	"Correct"

Thus, an individual or a situation can be "medicalized" when either should not have been (by the standards of modern medicine) or can fail to be "medicalized" when one or the other should have been. Both of these constitute "errors."

If a person or situation is medicalized, sociologically does it matter whether or not an error occurred? In a sense, it may not because many of the consequences would be the same, such as excusing the individual from other obligations and attempts at rehabilitation, for example. In another sense, it does make a difference but particularly as decisions about "correct" or "incorrect" medicalization are made by different participants to the process. If following medicalization it is "discovered" or believed that an error occurred, then additional consequences ensue. There emerges relief by the victim that he or she is not ill, anger and hostility toward the agents who made the error, a loss of confidence in the medicalizing agents, and a humbling of those who erred.

As indicated above, in modern industrial society there exists a set of occupations (with individuals trained to fill those statuses) that have as a major obligation the role of medicalizing. These are physicians, nurses, and others in similar positions. Some are engaged to a greater degree in initiating the medicalizing process, whereas others such as rehabilitation personnel are more oriented to dealing with the consequences of medicalization, that is, processing those who have already been medicalized and thereby embellishing the initial medicalization.

We should further note that in a society in which medicalizing is a legitimate activity, everyone engages in medicalizing. That is, nearly all individuals engage in creating medical explanations and interpretations of their own and others' behavior. Thus, the physician usually does not medicalize others in an arbitrary or random way. Rather, the physician completes a process begun by others. The patient by coming to the physician has already begun the process of self-medicalization.

SIGNIFICATION PROCESSES

Medicalization is but one of a number of what could be called "signification processes" — processes whereby members of a society create and assign shared meanings to the acts of members of that society. These meanings and interpretations depend on and reflect the values and beliefs of members of society. Thus, their interpretations will vary from society to society.

Another "signification process" is "criminalization." The former occurs more frequently, and with perhaps greater social significance, than the latter. In criminalization, individuals, because of some deviant behavior, are defined as (and may come to define self as) "delinquent," "criminal," "ne'er-do-well," "black sheep," "no-good," and the like. Ones who are so defined may simply characterize themselves as "losers," which is protective, because it implies they are only partly to blame; they have a vague belief that society (i.e., those with whom they have interacted) is also partly to blame. An example of this process is the case of the 12-year-old boy who hangs around a newsstand reading comics; one day he walks off with two comic books and is apprehended by the owner who calls the police. Because the boy may have a quasi-belligerent attitude, he is perceived by the owner and by police as a delinquent. His parents are called, and because they see his actions as causing them trouble and disrepute, also adopt and convey the label. "If you don't watch your step, you'll end up in reform school," they warn him. As with all 12 year olds, he has some doubts and questions about his identity;

he begins to think of himself as "troublesome." This image may affect his changing selection of peers, which further reinforces the image held of him by others, because his peers are others also seen as "troublesome." Thus, slowly and gradually an image develops that is related to behavior that is increasingly and more seriously rule-breaking and law-breaking; and thus, the process of criminalization has occurred.

The question is, of course: how frequently does this process occur? For this we have no evidence. But few would assert that it has never happened. A related question is: for each of those in jail, to what degree did this process of criminalization go on? Again, we have no evidence, but it is conceivable that it occurs to some degree in every instance. Some sociologists would have us believe that the response to an individual's initial mildly deviant act is the crucial factor that generates more severe deviant acts and a criminal career; the crucial factor is not any putative criminal nature or inclination to commit criminal acts.

LABELING PROCESSES

Several social processes (or happenings) have been described. These were referred to as "medicalization" and "criminalization" – and more generically, "signification processes." Within signification processes, but not identical to them, are "labeling processes." The labeling model of deviant behavior is shown below:

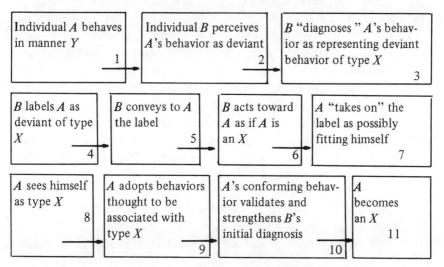

All that is necessary for the labeling process to occur, in this sequence of steps, is that (1) *A* be suggestible; (2) *A* and *B* be in sustained interaction; and (3) there exists no independent means to validate or refute the "diagnosis," or if they exist they are not utilized.

The diagram shown above is general and abstract. For *A*, *B*, *X*, and *Y*, different specific people, types, and behaviors can be inserted. Some possibilities are shown below:

A	B	Y	X
Son	Mother	Steals comic books	Delinquency
Wife	Husband	Is depressed	Mental disorder
Patient	Doctor	Chest pains	Cardiac patient
Patient	Psychiatrist	Withdrawn from interactions	Schizophrenic

Several things can be noted. In the first place, individual *B* may, in fact, be several individuals working in concert but not necessarily collusively. Thus, it might be family members and friends who define the wife's depression as signifying a mental disorder. Second, some individuals, and particularly the skillful and sensitive physician, recognizes the possibility of the process and hence aborts the process by not conveying in any direct fashion the label. Thus, some physicians who detect mild cardiac symptoms will "play down" their meaning to the patient while at the same time trying to get the patient to alter his or her life-style. The degree to which physicians do this may depend on their judgment about how suggestible the patient is.

Third, for this process to go to completion requires, as I have indicated, that *A* and *B* be in sustained interaction. As the ethnomethodologists remind us, if *A* and *B* are strangers to each other, and if *Y* is some nonthreatening but seemingly bizarre behavior, then *B* typically reverts to one of two diagnoses: *A* is either crazy or is making a sexual response. Ethnomethodologists note that members of any society interpret behavior and interactions in the light of their overall ideology or world view. That is, as members of a society each of us constructs order out of the social world. We cannot tolerate ambiguity or contemplate the possibility that the social world is random or chaotic or disorderly. We "explain" the bizarre behavior of another in order that our world and our experiences make sense; we do not believe that the bizarre behavior of another is unexplainable and just is. It must be bizarre because of something, and that something alters its bizarreness.

Fourth, this labeling process also describes to some degree personality formation. If A is an infant who has "colic" and B is A's mother, then B may define A as a cranky and difficult baby and act toward A as if A were a difficult child; over time, as A develops a personality and a sense of self, A comes to think of this self as difficult. This becomes a part of A's personality.

One question, then, is: to what degree is medicalization an instance of the labeling process? The labeling process connotes that sustained (as opposed to accidental and first-time) deviant behavior, whether sickness, mental disorder, or crime, is prolonged or fixed by the label being assigned to a deviant individual. To the degree that medicalization involves or results in a new social role, then to that degree the labeling process may have occurred. But medicalization is, in one sense, more than labeling and, in another sense, less than labeling.

The part of medicalization that is not labeling is the mere medicalizing of some happening or event. If individual A has stomach pains, goes to a physician, has an appendectomy, and returns to work after a few days, the social consequences of this have been fairly minor; no labeling has occurred.

That part of medicalization that is labeling is the case that results in a new role, a new self-image, and the like. That part of labeling that is not medicalizing is the labeling of behavior as something other than illness.

COUVADE AND MEDICALIZATION

Now let us turn to couvade and medicalization. From his study of the Bimin-Kuskusmin, a preliterate group of about 1,000 people living in highland New Guinea, Poole describes an elaborate set of behaviors that occur in husbands beginning when the pregnancy of their wives is evident and continuing through the first few weeks of life of the child. Lipkin discusses the emergence of what he calls the couvade condition, which includes symptoms of nausea, vomiting, constipation, and similar features, in 267 husbands of pregnant wives in a Rochester, New York, health center. Gabriel describes weight changes that occurred in a sample of 53 husbands she studied in Rochester.

The couvade refers to various "abnormal" behaviors that are observed to occur in the father around the time of the birth of his child. By "abnormal" is simply meant noteworthy or standing out in contrast to behaviors exhibited at other times. Furthermore, in some instances, the behaviors are believed to be intimately connected with the wife's pregnancy and subsequent delivery; and, the behaviors frequently imitate or simulate the physiological responses of the woman to her pregnancy — although it is possible that those responses could be culturally induced and not totally physiological. Among those responses are nausea, vomiting, and abdominal pain.

This definition is confined to the physical and emotional distress felt and expressed by the father on the occasion of his wife's pregnancy and delivery; it excludes nonphysiological behaviors that may co-occur with the pregnancy, such as avoiding certain foods or avoiding the taro garden, as described by Poole in Chapter 5. That is, in every society there may be a number of elaborately developed customs associated with pregnancy and birth; these are expected of those who are party to it, such as the baby showers or cigar-giving that occur in the United States.

Thus, couvade has four elements that jointly set it off from other phenomena; these are (1) "physiological behaviors"; (2) behaviors that are "abnormal" (such as weight loss or vomiting); (3) behaviors that "occur in the father"; and (4) behaviors that occur "around the time of the wife's pregnancy and delivery."

Although there is a unitary thing such as couvade, as defined above, there are different forms of it — as revealed in the previous three chapters. Two types that can be distinguished are: (1) idiosyncratic or individual couvade (as described in the chapters by Gabriel and Lipkin) and (2) customary or ritual couvade (as described by Poole). The former occurs randomly, and those men exhibiting the behavior are usually not aware of its connection to their wives' pregnancy. The latter occurs more frequently; it is expected of the husbands and is sustained by some form of sanctions. Participants are aware of the tie with pregnancy.

This raises the question: what are the mechanisms that generate couvade? It would appear that the mechanisms differ for these two forms of couvade. Ritual or customary couvade is learned, as are other customs. Men understand what behavior is appropriate for them when they are in the position of expectant father. But this is not the case for idiosyncratic couvade. There the causal mechanism is more complex.

COUVADE IN AN ANALYSIS OF ILLNESS: OBJECTIVE STATE OR PERCEPTION

It may be that illness should be analyzed in terms of its occurrence and the perception of its occurrence, namely, the difference between the presence or absence of illness, in some objective sense, and the belief that illness is present or absent; these two do not necessarily coincide. Furthermore, for the case of an illness being present, it is useful to distinguish between socially caused illness and biologically caused illness. This can be represented in the following diagram:

		An objectively defined pathological condition is		
		Present		Absent
		Cause:		
		Social	Biological	
It is believed that the condition is:	Present	I	II	III
	Absent	IV	V	VI

Thus, we have distinguished six cases. It may be problematic whether a pathological condition can be "objectively" discerned as present: we assume that in theory it can be, although in practice it may be difficult. For example, *in the extreme*, a condition called rheumatic fever can be objectively identified; that is, for a "classic" case, an individual with all of the textbook symptoms, there would be no disagreement among trained observers who proceed from different perspectives that individual X has all the abnormal physiological features called rheumatic fever. This would be case II. Alternatively, an individual may be, say, "prediabetic," in that some of the signs are present (e.g., extreme thirst) but that some are absent (e.g., lack of excessive urination). Such an individual may, in fact, be diabetic but, given the present diagnostic techniques, this is not clearly evident to physicians. At some point the condition is suspected but not definitely confirmed; or prior to any visit to a doctor, there is no perception or belief that individual *Y* is diabetic. This, then, would be shown by case V in our diagram above.

Just as it may be difficult to ascertain that a particular disease condition is present in a particular individual, it is equally or more difficult to determine its cause. Clearly, many diseases have both a biological and a social cause. For example, individual *Z* contracts malaria; the cause is the parasite transmitted to *Z* by a mosquito. However, there may be a social cause in the factors that led *Z* to be where the mosquito could inflict the bite. At the other extreme are diseases that *some think* are largely socially induced, such as ulcers or asthma. Again, we can distinguish the perceptions that such disorders are present or absent.

Where does couvade fit into this analytical scheme? In the first place, it seems clear that it represents socially caused pathological conditions that may or may not be recognized as present (i.e., cases I or IV). Among the Bimin-Kuskusmin of New Guinea there is no such notion of something being pathological, although they may recognize behavior as being "out-of-the-ordinary." That a husband truly is anorexic or suffers from abdominal cramps is not considered abnormal in this setting but could be seen by Western observers as objectively pathological. If he showed these behaviors when his wife was not pregnant, he and others might see them as different and "out-of-the-ordinary," attributing the behavior to evil spirits that need to be exorcised. However, he is expected to show such behaviors when his wife is pregnant. Thus, the Bimin-Kuskusmin clearly see these behaviors as necessarily tied to the occasion of pregnancy and delivery.

On the other hand, the men in Rochester, as observed by Gabriel and Lipkin and Lamb, seem largely unaware that their pregnancy-like behavior was initiated by their wives' pregnancy (although some of the husbands in Gabriel's study apparently lost weight deliberately, under the rationale that their child needed a healthy father). Thus, there may be some "unconscious" mental mechanism interceding between two observable behaviors; that is, the pregnancy of the wife has some psychological effect on the husband that is not directly evident (for example, it is not evident in his own self-awareness as represented by a statement like "I was worried about whether the baby would be healthy") but rather indirectly evident in behavior such as nausea and vomiting.

Couvade, then, would appear to be an instance of behavior of categories I and IV; in ritual couvade, it is type I, and with idiosyncratic couvade, it is type IV, and in some cases type I.

COUVADE AND LABELING

Finally, we will briefly consider whether the couvade is an instance of the labeling process. The labeling process, sometimes referred to as the "societal reaction theory," has been used above as an explanation for some forms of pathological behavior.

It is clear that pregnancy is not a label assigned to women, which in turn causes them to be pregnant. A wife who is not pregnant may be nauseated and show other signs suggesting pregnancy; her husband or mother may say to her, "You are pregnant," and she may believe it — by buying maternity clothes and other behavior. But in two or three months, unequivocal signs must be evident or the label will not persist. Thus, pregnancylike behavior might emerge in a woman who labels herself as pregnant, but that behavior is of short duration.

In a like fashion, pregnancylike behavior in husbands may result in part from the labeling process, but this occurs only in societies in which such behavior is expected. That is, when his wife is pregnant, a Bimin-Kuskusmin husband knows that he is supposed to show pregnancylike behavior. He is labeled "husband-of-a-mother-to-be." As such, the knowledge of what is expected may be a powerful suggestion and a powerful cause of that behavior. Thus, the labeling process, or something like it, may be the mechanism that generates the couvade in societies in which the couvade is traditional or ritual behavior. However, in societies such as the United States, the couvade occurs, if at all, not because of labeling but by virtue of some other processes. What those processes are remain to be elucidated.

REFERENCES

Becker, H. S. 1973. *Outsiders*. New York: Free Press.

Conrad, P. 1976. *Identifying Hyperactive Children: The Medicalization of Deviant Behavior*. Lexington, Mass.: D. C. Heath.

Conrad, P., and Schneider, J. W. 1980. *Deviance and Medicalization: From Badness to Sickness*. St. Louis: Mosby.

Gove, W. R., ed. 1980. *The Labeling of Deviance*. Beverly Hills, Calif.: Sage.

Lemert, E. M. 1972. *Human Deviance, Social Problems and Social Control*. Englewood Cliffs, N.J.: Prentice-Hall.

_____. 1951. *Social Pathology*. New York: McGraw-Hill.

Scheff, T. J. 1966. *Being Mentally Ill*. Chicago: Aldine.

Schur, E. M. 1971. *Labeling Deviant Behavior*. New York: Harper & Row.

_____. 1979. *Interpreting Deviance*. New York: Harper & Row.

9

DISEASE AND ILLNESS AS PROCESSES:
The Lessons of the Couvade Example for a Notion of Appropriate Medical Care

Mack Lipkin, Jr.

What are medicine's functions and how satisfactorily are they discharged? This chapter represents an effort in clinical reasoning to examine this root question about medical care. It uses the example of couvade in Rochester presented in Chapter 6 to sketch the sequence of events that occurs in a typical case of couvade syndrome. It then examines what this sequence of events shows about the nature of illness episodes and the labeling and care processes. This leads to hypotheses about the relationships of labeling, clinical reasoning, and clinical decisions and their relations to medicine's functions. This is relevant to the question of medicalization because medicalization can be defined as the inappropriate extension of medicine beyond its appropriate limits of function.

I approach this question differently than those who for personal, social, or political reasons are interested to expose medicine's odious tendencies. Medical criticism has a welcome and useful function. It can cleanse, purify, and redirect. But criticism that is rhetorical or excessively general can actually contribute to the trends it fears or denounces. The spirit of my inquiry is not that of a social critic. Nor is it that of a medical accuser or defender. It is that of a person engaged in medical practice and puzzled in the attempt to provide more comfort and to do less harm to those coming in pain for relief of suffering. In this process questions of what is appropriate care often arise. I have seen patients be treated well and also be misunderstood, misdiagnosed, and mistreated. In addition, I have seen the medical system burdened to the point of breaking. I have seen colleagues burn out, tune out, cop out, and drop out. The critics are right that something is wrong. The pilot couvade study described in Chapter 6 was undertaken in an attempt to get a handle on a small aspect of this problem and has contributed to a broader analysis.

I make certain assumptions. First, I assume that the reader is familiar with the prior chapters in this section. The material presented here will make no sense without understanding couvade. Second, I make an intellectual assumption about the notion of sequence. The idea of sequence is a heuristic. The descriptive units selected to denote a sequence are always arbitrary. They do, however, reveal some of the things of interest or importance to the describer of the sequence. This is the problem of a riverboat pilot attempting to describe the course of the river: whereas the river flows continuously, one picks out river landmarks — often beside, beneath, or above it — that have special significance in getting downstream. Similarly, I conceptualize illness events as part of a constant flow in which biological, psychological, and social boundaries interact continuously.

SEQUENCE IN COUVADE

In this section the events that occur in a typical illness episode of couvade in Rochester, New York, will be described. Although we are discussing a specific, arbitrary episode, each episode has both phylogenetic and ontogenetic history: the individuals involved in an episode have a prior history together and separately. As well, intra- and interspecies evolution may play significant roles. I mention these because illness experience is part of evolutionary processes not unique to humans.

However, in an illness episode of couvade the first step is that an ovum is fertilized, a woman bears a conceptus, and physical changes occur in her. These physical changes include hormonal changes such as increased progesterone; organ changes such as swelling of the breasts and abdomen and softening of the cervix; psychological changes such as increased self-concern, increase in appetite, and changes in libido; and behavioral changes such as starting to get the house in order and developing new (and sometimes strange) eating habits.

Somewhere along this line, a cognitive change occurs. A woman becomes aware that she has missed her menses and considers whether or not she is pregnant. In some cases this is cause for joy; in others, alarm. Some women know this early on in conception, and others do not know until the last days. In every such event the woman has feelings and attitudes toward the possibility that she may be pregnant.

Once these feelings and attitudes develop the woman may or may not take action concerning them. In particular, she may or may not seek confirmation of the biological fact of pregnancy. Some ignore, some deny, some wait to see, some talk to their mate about this, some keep him in the dark, and some get a pregnancy test.

If a woman in Rochester going to our health maintenance organization wants a pregnancy test, she obtains an appointment, keeps it, gives a history, has a physical, provides a urine sample, and waits for the results. She is informed of the results. Usually at this point the woman's feelings and attitudes are mixed and complicated.

At the same time, both because she is the bearer of a physical change and is typically in control of the information about it, significant changes occur in the couple. (Note how arbitrary this sequence has become.) The husband may or may not have noticed or be concerned about any of the changes, feelings, or attitudes mentioned above. The couple may or may not have discussed her bodily changes. She may or may not be showing changes or acting differently. There may be sexual differences or subliminal differences such as pheromonal differences. The man will have his own feelings and attitudes about these things, separately and together.

All these events lead, then, to some changes in the mate of the pregnant woman. He may have reactions to any or all of them. These reactions will be determined by his prior personal history as well as by his genetics. His attitudes about her, his feelings about pregnancy, and his life context and situation will each influence the feelings and attitudes he develops. In particular, he may have complex psychological changes — feelings of joy, despair, loss, pride. He may have reactive and complex physiological changes, including increased growth hormone, increased cortisone production, and changes in appetite, weight, or libido. He may have complex psychophysiological changes such as release of endorphins. In addition, he may have changes in self-perception.

In those men who experience couvade, their self-perception changes. They experience a sense that something physically is wrong. This may be a pain, a sense of something being inappropriate, a discomfort, or something harder to put into words than that. Such a man evaluates the severity and potential significance of what he is experiencing. He decides whether or not to seek care. If he decides not to seek care, he may do so later or he may undertake some self-treatment. In deciding to seek care he makes decisions about the appropriate source of care based on his perception of the problem, his perception of the potential solution, and his situation and prior history (Mechanic, 1972).

If he seeks care he encounters the physician who elicits data actively (history). The physician also notes cues (physical). From these sources the physician generates hypotheses about the nature of the problem and tests these hypotheses by historical or physical examination or by laboratory tests. Then some or all of these test results are analyzed in accordance with the physician's specialty or some other trained or cultural or intuitive classificatory paradigms. A problem or diagnosis is identified: this then allows the physician to carry out the steps that are perceived as necessary (through training, intuition, or other predilections, or for personal satisfaction) to test the validity of the problem and diagnostic choices. The physician proceeds to diagnose further, to confirm diagnosis, or to treat, with or without diagnosis. The physician's views of the problems are modified, and further steps are taken in stepwise, possibly Bayesian, fashion. Communication with the patient about what is to be done and how to do it is undertaken.

The patient chooses how to deal with the doctor's findings and perceptions and with the issues of how he feels about what he has been told. He chooses how to communicate with his present mate about these proceedings.

A man who simply *experiences* symptoms and does not seek care is considered to have couvade *condition*. A man who *seeks care* for the symptoms and has them associated with the pregnancy has couvade *syndrome*.

LABELING AND COUVADE

The above sketch highlights some of the interlocked events that become condensed into the description that a patient has couvade condition or couvade syndrome. The question then arises: is such a description of such a complex event, such labeling either by patient and/or physician, appropriate?

That of course depends on outcomes to some extent, but it also depends on many other notions about the nature of illness as a process, the reality of diseases and disease labels, and one's assessment of the relationship between the act of labeling and identification and subsequent events of care.

In the couvade example the sequence of events helps us to identify some of the elements in the confusion about labeling. The first events in the episode involve the wife. Next, internal disturbances in her mate derived from unspecified and uncertain stimuli from the pregnant woman led from the experience of sensation in the mate to his perception of it as abnormal. After diagnostic processes involving the doctor's thinking and history-taking and then doing tests, the men became variously labeled in Rochester as carriers of things. Specifically they acquired such labels as "peptic ulcer syndrome" and "dyspepsia." Such labels do not alter the sequence of events or change their prior nature, although labels have subsequent effects. The designation of a person as having couvade syndrome would not change the prior realities of his history but would effect further diagnostic and treatment steps.

Yet this act of labeling concerns many, such as Harper in Chapter 8. By labeling, I mean, as do most who write about labeling, a process by which a person becomes identified professionally or personally as suffering from a specific defined entity, whether it is a professional definition or a lay definition. This assumes that several important prior steps have occurred that are often not defined or clarified in discussions of labeling (Locker, 1980). First, the person who is suffering has to identify that suffering. Second, that person has to identify him/herself as a patient or a potential patient. This is done by seeking care. Third, the patient must submit to some process that makes professional labeling possible, by submitting to an examination through which the attachment of the label is justified. It is through such processes that patient characteristics become identified. Some of the debates about labeling have to do with the philosophical aspects of the process of *identification* of patient characteristics. The next step is *matching* of the patient's characteristics to a label through the use of a classification.

The example of couvade in Rochester is instructive concerning labeling. Identification of the patients' characteristics, through the acquisition of historical and laboratory data was clearly flawed. The physicians responsible for identification of the patient character-istics *did not* often elicit the relevant psychosocial datum of the wife's pregnancy. Thus, they were unable to make an appropriate match of characteristics and diagnosis or label (if they knew the label). The chances that their label would be correct were dimin-ished. This is a case in which the failure is one of *too narrow* rather than too broad a set of investigations.

A second set of concerns regarding labeling has to do with feeling that the label itself may harm patients either by stigmatizing them or by in some way diminishing their self-image. Harper's discus-sion of this in Chapter 8, however, crucially omits recognition or acceptance of the prior step of the patient choosing to seek care as a result of his identified suffering. These arguments fail to recognize that the responsibility for elicitation of the characteristics of the patient and for the matching of characteristics to the label sets rests neither primarily nor exclusively with the physician. Critics often fall into the fallacy that physicians are exclusively responsible to "take a history" and fail to recognize that the patient is equally responsible to "give a history." In this, the ability of each to find the appropriate data depends on one's own sense of what "appropriate" is. This is the main focus of this exercise. The couvade example clearly demonstrates that the omitted psychosocial data are relevant. Paradigms for *both* patients and physicians may be lacking.

Arguments for holistic medicine often center on this issue. They state that if patients could be more involved in the creation and identification of the characteristics pool and the label-matching process, more accuracy of labeling might result. The problem, of course, is in the creation of patients able to do such matching. There is an interaction between patient and physician in which they mutually determine the pooled characteristics to be considered. The pool of characteristics sought by physicians are often too limited, as in the couvade example. As well, their label sets may also be too limited. But certainly as well, the same problems may exist with patients. Both groups share a paradigm that is too limited!

Finally, there is a complex of concerns about the issue of reifica-tion, the conceptual error of confusing the label with the real thing in nature. There is the fear that if a person is labeled the person will actually become a carrier of something. There is a fear that it is dangerous to label something that has complex relationships with normal phenomena because the normality of the thing labeled may become lost to view and it may be seen as sick or distinct. Since some such experiences, such as couvade, might be seen as extensions, exaggerations, or outer limits of normal life cycle events, should they be called syndromes or given disease labels? The bottom line is that the person who determines whether this will occur in fact is not the physician but the patient. The patient is the one who experiences self as abnormal and seeks care for the abnormality. However, it is the physician's responsibility to correctly identify the nature of the problem and, when it is an extension of the normal, to deal with it as such, rather than to bring the patient into new realms of needless dependency.

In this example, problems with defining a disease become apparent. First is the existence of numerous sets of analytical distinctions dependent on language, culture, point of view (e.g., patient, physician, third party payer), classificatory persuasion (e.g., anatomical, physiological, problem oriented), and most of all the use to which the distinction is to be put. Common usage in the sociological and anthropological sense uses "illness" to denote the subjective or person-centered aspects of the sequence of events. "Disease" denotes the objective aspects. The definition of "objective" varies. Usually it refers not only to those things that are tested by external laboratory instruments but also to the use of the physician as an "objective" instrument. (This is despite large quantities of data that intraobserver reliability in physician assessments is extremely variable.)

It is also apparent that the distinctions of disease and illness in common use are insufficient to handle or disentangle the sequence of events described above. I would prefer to use a single term when possible and to view whichever term is used, be it "disease" or "illness," as a process. It seems sensible to include in the definition of a disease those elements of the sequence of events that contribute to the experience of abnormal sensation and that contribute to any other set of evaluatory functions that lead to recognition of a state of abnormality whether this is detected through personal (i.e., sensory in the patient), indirect (i.e., through the physician's taking of a history or doing an examination), or impersonal (laboratory sensing) means. In this view, disease consists of a procession of events that can be detected sometimes subjectively and sometimes through testing. The disease is then never solely limited to those manifestations of the process that happen to be measured by the instruments at hand.

A second set of problems about disease and labels is the existence of noxious tangles of attitudes about the decision to call something a disease. These are the ancient problems of the reality of denotation and the charged quality of connotation. Thus, some regard a disease as something that could be autopsied or measured. All else to them is scientific nonsense. Others confuse the uses of a classification with abuses of it. Brown does this in Chapter 15 in this book. Some medicalization critics such as Szasz feel that to call something a disease renders the carrier of it subject to abuses better avoided by avoiding labeling altogether.

It seems more sensible to recognize that labeling is potentially subject to *abuse* of various sorts as well as to *error* of various sorts. Then it follows that one ought to label only when it serves a useful purpose, when the reliability is known, and when the potential for good outweighs the potential for harm.

To apply such decision rules about labeling, we need to identify, measure, and weigh the benefits and harms of labeling. To do this requires the use of tracer or model conditions to study these benefits and harms. This is the contribution of the couvade example. It requires, also, an analytical approach to assessments, benefits, and harms and empirical techniques for their application. These are presently under development (Banta, 1982).

The couvade pilot study gave two examples of the effects of mislabeling. The first was that mislabels occurred that had implications for action that were, albeit mildly so, unfortunate. Thus, mislabeling led to performance of procedures and tests, prescriptions of potentially dangerous medications, and so forth. This sort of error is to some extent unavoidable. But it must be minimized since it produces needless morbidity and mortality and generates unnecessary costs that are both wasteful and divert resources from more beneficial use. Diversion of resources may lead secondarily to elevated morbidity and mortality.

The second effect of failure to label properly was loss of opportunity to help. This assumes that the condition involved can in some way be helped by appropriate identification and subsequent management (even if the management is to do nothing else but assure that no further steps are taken). Generally, proper labeling may in some cases lead to increased opportunity to help, although it need not necessarily do so. However, proper diagnosis is neither a necessary nor a sufficient condition of helping. Osler focused on diagnosis not to help but to teach. Often the greatest help is to take no action but to explain in culturally appropriate ways the value of inaction.

COUVADE AS AN EXAMPLE OF AN
ILLNESS-DISEASE PROCESS

There are some general aspects of the illness process that the couvade example highlights. It presents a situation in which the patient and the doctor each feel that what is going on is a physical process; yet we have found it most natural to describe it as a primary psychosocial process. To understand this better, a first query is what does the patient actually experience? Those couvade patients whom I have interviewed, and others in analogous situations, are very clear that their complaints are felt as physical. They are sensed in their bodies like other sensations. (Note that this, too, has its shades of gray — my patient, who suddenly felt concerned about a growth he had had for years, felt annoyance and anxiety rather than pain or discomfort.) If one avoids debates about solipsism (how can I know what you feel . . . am I right that I feel what I think I feel . . .), and if one remains agnostic about the issue of the interactions between suggestion, prior conceptual frame, and present perception of sensation (we usually feel what we expect or wish to feel, we experience only what we believe possible . . .), there still remains a desire to understand how this can come about. There is an extensive literature and some controversy on this subject. In my view, it is common for people to experience feelings indirectly. For example, some people experience feelings not directly as emotions, such as sadness or anger, but as bodily sensation, such as malaise or pain. The form the sensation takes is, in some cases, *symbolic* (e.g., a pain in the neck). In some cases, it can be *idiosyncratic* as in old sensations relived but disguised. In other cases, it may also be a cultural (or species) universal as in couvade. I believe it is not necessarily pathological to experience oneself thus. It may be adaptive or unadaptive depending on setting and point of view. But it is part of a sequence of events that must be managed or understood by someone hoping to help!

A second, separable set of cases involves the occasional occurrence of physical *signs* in reaction to feelings. An example is the increased abdominal protuberance in some men in couvade cases. This leads to exaggerated spinal curvature, which produces a secondary, mechanically induced, back pain.

A third mechanism was suggested to me by the case of a leading research scientist. He became troubled by hemorrhoidal pain and bleeding when his wife first became pregnant. He paid no attention to the relation of pregnancy and hemorrhoids until they occurred again during his wife's second and third pregnancies. They occurred only when she was pregnant, never in between. He convinced himself this was not coincidence when his hemorrhoids recurred during her fourth and fifth pregnancies. His children are now grown, and he has not had any recurrence of hemorrhoids. Here, psychophysiological events have intervened between the causal psychosocial change (the wife's pregnancy) and the development of pain and bleeding in the husband's perianal vasculature. That we cannot specify the psychophysiological chain does not alter our perception that a causal chain exists – it only places a portion of the sequence in a black box.

So we have three separate mechanisms. In the first the psychosocial event, without gross physiological change (i.e., with only the subtle physiological change associated with mind activity), results in sensation indistinguishable from garden-variety physical symptoms. Second, we have a mechanism in which minor physical alteration, in which the patient changes and looks more like his mate, leads to secondary symptom development. Third, we have obscure psychophysiological changes determining clear-cut pathological alteration (e.g., hemorrhoids) in a psychologically and physically vulnerable individual. Other types of psychosocial-physical interactions were not encountered in this example. These include, most importantly, alterations in homeostasis and/or in host resistance leading to increased susceptibility to some or another toxin, infection, imbalance, or illness (Cassel, 1976). Thus, for example, a member of a population has a greater probability of illness, any illness, at times of life change (Holmes and Rahe, 1967; Dohrenwend and Dohrenwend, 1974).

MULTIPLE CAUSAL CHAINS AS EXPLANATIONS OF ILLNESS

What I am suggesting here is that multiple mechanisms can account for the occurrence of causal chains from a psychological or social event to the development of illness behavior. Multiple events ensue in which the illness behavior is evaluated and altered by patient and health care personnel. In some, but not all cases, knowledge of the chain is needed to decide where to intervene. For some, but not all cases, knowledge of the chain is helpful. Thus, my patient with low back pain required discussion of pregnancy and then corrected his posture himself. The scientist with hemorrhoids sought and self-administered appropriate symptomatic care.

In the couvade situation, the most common patients are those in whom no apparent or important intervening psychophysiological or psychoanatomical alterations occur. Such patients mostly need protection from mislabeling and inappropriate diagnostic maneuvers or treatments. They tend to get better by themselves. If not, they continue to seek care until they either find appropriate discussion of their feelings or find a substitute relationship for what they are missing; here for what they lose in the pregnancy of their mate. (This is not to imply that they must or can find this through professional care in every case.) They probably represent a mild subset of those experiencing themselves in the complex interaction of body and mind that creates sensations for them instead of what are emotions for others. The provider who is unaware of this possibility, of how common it is, and of how to deal with it, or who lacks this concept or a name for it, mistakenly searches too diligently, expensively, and dangerously for pathology.

THE APPROPRIATE SEARCH FOR DATA

But what level of search is appropriate for which kind of data, to support which set of explanations, to help whom? Only clear answers to each of these questions can lead to sense about medicalization. Clearly, when a patient is suffering from psychological pain or social dislocation, data relevant to that may be relevant to the care of the patient. It is not medicalizing to elicit such data — it is being appropriate. This is because illness phenomena interact, through such mechanisms as described above, with all other human phenomena. This is not only a psychological or social phenomenon, it is a biological fact.

LABELING: CLINICAL DECISION MAKING

When the patient is suffering from a dominantly pathological or physiological ailment, it is appropriate to obtain data relevant both to it and to the precipitating factors. When there is not a precipitating psychological or social factor (which is a rare case), the only necessary data are anatomical and physiological. A practitioner cannot always know which sort of case one is encountering as the patient enters the room. This dilemma leads to the various forms of diagnostic search that characterize varied groups of health personnel. Some, not knowing what class of data will be helpful, attempt to fill all classes as exhaustively as possible. Some, caring mainly for one type of data (often related to a test or procedure for which they are trained or from which they profit academically or financially) search for it mainly. Some use cues in the interaction to guide them. The majority of clinical encounters are of the sort that uses cues. It is here that the labeling process is critical, because the cues used come from the same set of incorporated concepts as do labels.

This is especially important in view of the nature of clinical decision making. Seemingly, the majority of physicians use neither a modification of regression analysis in a computerized (or head-computerized) screening of probabilistic data nor the sort of differential diagnosis modeled in the clinicopathological conferences of the Massachusetts General Hospital. Rather, like most other humans they begin with a very few hypotheses, based on precious few cues, and test them (Elstein et al., 1978). Depending on the probabilistic match of their repertoire of hypotheses (i.e., concepts and labels) and tests to the nature of their practice population, and their flexibility and openness to considering alternative hypotheses (which relates to their tolerance for ambiguity), they may get more or less close to accurate solutions.

Given how clinicians proceed, the solutions they settle for will be limited to a subset of the universe of hypotheses they can generate. This is why their initial disease models and paradigms are critical. How clinicians decide also explains the circular insularity of the present resistance to consideration of the role of psychosocial factors in the generation and maintenance of illness. A hypothesis seldom generated will seldom be proved correct and hence will seldom be perceived to be important or prevalent. This will decrease its probability of generation in later cases (Bayes' theorem). Lists of what is common are only as complete as their initial category classes. Similarly, clinicians' views of what things commonly relate to one another are subject to the initial cues and categories to which they respond and to the hypotheses they generate. If you do not name and record it, you cannot count it. If it is not counted, it does not count.

CONCLUSIONS

These considerations lead to several conclusions. Many common problems may not be recognized at all because they are not in the current sets of hypotheses generated by clinicians and counters of care. Failure to realize the possible mechanisms involving psychosocial factors and their relations to illness and disease may cause them not to be tested for or to be tested for incorrectly.

So the education of practitioners should include exercises leading to incorporated awareness of the entire variety of mechanisms relevant in the development of illness behavior and disease processes. This must reach the level of effecting the sets of hypotheses they generate in response to physical illness cues.

Second, the sets of data from which we derive our concepts of what is prevalent and what is rare, what is important and what is trivial, must be expanded to allow us to assess new sorts of conditions, call them what they are, and learn how to help those who experience them as safely and as well as possible.

To accomplish this expansion, more research into the multifactorial determinants of each of the links in the chain of events sketched here, and many other such chains, must be accomplished. There doubtless exist illness conditions for each of the life cycle events of humanity. These are yet to be described systematically. There are doubtless illness conditions for the common crises of humanity. A goal is to come to recognize these on the basis of clinically practical cues. This could abort the expensive and dangerous idealized course of the exhaustive search of all possible categories, which is only available to the rich anyway. At present we see, instead, arbitrary compulsive searches of arbitrary subsets of possibilities based on the idiosyncratic preferences of practitioner and patient.

The medicalization issue in this analysis reduces to questions of what is appropriate and when. More appropriate diagnostic and evaluative skills must be based on more complete models. A new science of clinical epidemiology that shows the true prevalence of the full range of conditions in the specified population under treatment is needed. Each region and culture will have to evolve its own subset of data on the nature and distribution of specific illnesses, but universal principals and mechanisms may also be elaborated. This can be the basis for increased humanization of care, which is the implicit goal of some of those who now object to the extension of dehumanized medical systems.

I have argued here that appropriate medical care is congruent with humanistic medical care, not because of the hopes of well-meaning scholars but because of the nature of illness and wellness.

REFERENCES

Banta, D. 1982. *Resources for Health: Technology Assessment for Policy Making*. New York: Praeger.

Cassel, J. 1976. The Contributions of the Social Environment to Host Resistance. *Am. J. Epidemiol.* 104(2):107-23.

Dohrenwend, B., and Dohrenwend, B. 1974. *Stressful Life Events: Their Nature and Effects*. New York: Wiley.

Elstein, A.; Shulman, L. S.; and Sprafa, S. A. 1978. *Medical Problem Solving*. Cambridge, Mass.: Harvard University Press.

Holmes, T., and Rahe, R. 1967. Social Readjustment Rating Scale. *J. Psychosom. Res.* 11:213-18.

Locker, D. 1980. *Symptoms and Illness*. London: Tavistock.

Mechanic, D. 1972. Social Psychologic Factors Affecting the Presentation of Bodily Complaints. *N. Engl. J. Med.* 286:1132-39.

PART III

Organizing Around the Fact of Illness

The previous chapters have described a series of contextual views of medicalization and have shown how the nature of the illness process may justify a concept of medicalization that includes both normative and descriptive elements. That is, one can both describe how medicine interfaces with other elements of society and ask about the described interactions in what senses they are appropriate or not. The couvade example illustrates that the dominant problem in modern Western medicine may not be its expansionism or aggrandizement but its inappropriate models. Both in the interaction of the Bimin-Kuskusmin and in the Western couvade condition, a broader, more integrative model would permit more appropriate care.

The authors in the following section look at a second aspect of the processes of health and illness — those in which providers of care get involved in therapeutic interactions, in the organization of care, and in their training and socialization for care.

In Chapter 10, Janzen makes several arguments relevant to broader considerations of the proper role of medicine. In his description of the drums anonymous, he makes a striking synthesis of diverse groups in cultures from slaving tribal Africa to the modern (post Vietnam) Plains Indians to urban alcoholics in Alcoholics Anonymous. He shows that these groups draw together people suddenly experiencing helplessness with a common affliction. Their drawing together provides them with social support, new status, and sometimes new wealth or power somehow reframing this experience from that of suffering to a virtue. He has discovered in his cross-cultural work a system-wide principle of healing analogous to reframing and paradoxical intention psychotherapy techniques. Additionally, he illustrates that most cultures possess healing mechanisms

151

outside their explicit and orthodox medical system with considerable potential for helping. He notes in passing that these groups have economic implications and that because they involve patients, they resist takeover by orthodox providers. For example, Alcoholics Anonymous is not used by physicians in the United States except as a referral aid. Janzen's argument has relevance to the medicalization critique because it posits the existence of multiple modes of healing in most societies and illustrates their complexity in a way that causes one to resist simplistic descriptions of single healing modalities. At the same time, he illustrates both positive and negative aspects of the drums he describes.

A second way to look at how therapeutic services are integrated or not in a society is to examine how it is regulated and governed. Berg, in Chapter 11, succinctly summarizes how the government of Yugoslavia has evolved a system of health governance that emphasizes local control through a democratic process. The local planners are elected and have a single pot of resources to work with. Thus, any increases in medical services must come from some other source, and it is hard to create creeping medicalization under such careful scrutiny. He notes, however, that there is informal correction of this system through a secret economy of bribes and influence that lubricates the overt system's function. Again, the descriptive approach leads to a view that social mechanisms can be used to control medicalization.

In Chapter 12, Ross takes this consideration several steps further in a conceptual essay that attempts to sketch some of the social aspects of medical acculturation both of patients and providers of health care. Viewing culture as the structuring of information, she shows that it is the rule that multiple rather than unitary strategies exist for getting care and that cultures, even primitive or small ones, have a hierarchical approach to seeking care. Thus, no single system can be expected to take over since the normal cultural pattern is to have multiple parallel systems operant. In Western cultures, in addition to allopathic medicine, there coexist chiropractors, osteopaths, faith healers, root healers, and so forth. Ross then illustrates other aspects of medical-cultural interactions, including the influence of past arrangements such as body snatching on the present-day system. She asserts, for example, that the early training experience of working with cadavers conditions the future physicians to think in terms of cross-sectional phenomena (omitting the element of time absent in the cadaver) and to expect the patient to be passive as is the corpse.

The principal means of socialization of practitioners is through their training. Pfifferling looks in depth at the process of becoming a physician in the United States in Chapter 13 and describes the many ways that the education and training are also socializing and, even, he asserts, brainwashing. Students are made subservient, their time is controlled, and they are dressed in rigid fashion, exhausted, humiliated, and constantly pushed to the dogmatic behaviors of the care institution. This process of medicalizing of the person is sketched more personally in Chapter 14 by Schiffer, who highlights some of his own experiences in the noncognitive parts of becoming a physician. Both Pfifferling and Schiffer clearly demonstrate the depth of this process and imply that its impact on the medical student and resident is enormous.

10

DRUMS ANONYMOUS:
Toward an Understanding of
Structures of Therapeutic Maintenance

John M. Janzen

DEFINITION OF DRUMS ANONYMOUS

What do sufferers of scrotal hernias, parents of twins, those who have nightmares of their oppressors, the nouveau riche of seventeenth century Congo coastal trading routes, urban isolated women, Plains warriors returned from war with nothing to do, alcoholics, child abusing parents, drug addicts, heart attack victims, and organ donors and recipients and their relatives have in common? On a cross-cultural basis, sufferers of these modes of affliction have been brought from the isolation of their sickness together with others of the same affliction and have given each other mutual support to reenter society, indeed, even to become specialized healers of their affliction. In Africa, among Bantu societies south of the rain forests, such organizations are called "drums of affliction." In the Plains of North America, Indian societies speak of the genre as "dance societies." In Euroamerican society they are called "X, Y, and Z Anonymous." Thus, I refer to them as "drums . . . anonymous." Their common characteristics are so striking that it is worthwhile to explore them as representatives of a much larger class of therapeutic maintenance units for a host of chronic afflictions. I shall briefly describe each example in my sample of drums anonymous and then analyze their common characteristics.

154

EXAMPLES OF DRUMS ANONYMOUS

The Pende of Kasai region of Zaire before the advent of Western surgery, in about 1930, used to have what they called the "chiefship of the scrotal hernia." The Pende are active hunters and traders for whom a scrotal hernia is normally a severe handicap. At some point in the past the sufferers of this affliction asserted themselves so as to receive the recognition of other leaders in their society. A concept and a political entity coalesced into a chiefly order, transforming these individuals who were physically incapacitated, but otherwise perfectly intelligent, into an order of chiefs who got involved in judicial affairs; they became, in effect, sitting judges of the "chiefship of the scrotal hernia," an important, positive institution (De Sousberghe, 1958).

In many parts of Africa parents of twins are similarly recognized, and in the southern savanna, the Lunda region, a drum of affliction has been developed in most societies for parents of twins and twinship. Turner has evolved a long analysis on Wubwangu, the twin cult among the Ndembu. You find also twins, parents of twins, and twinship being recognized among the West African people, such as the Yoruba of Nigeria and the BaKongo of Lower Zaire. According to Turner, twins are significant for a variety of reasons, both metaphysical and physical. In Central African cosmological thinking, duality is one step removed from ultimate unity; thus duality represents the conceptual transition from the one to the many, the same problem that concerned ancient Greek philosophers (Turner, 1969). Twinship, just as the androgynous hero, the set of siblings, or any other natural duality, is grist for the philosophical mill about conceptual duality. Twins really are difficult to handle. Identical twins can be especially problematic. They move around like a unit; yet you have to respond to them as two individuals. They are one, and yet they are two. Thus the Central African twinship drums bring together parents of twins on a local basis for the appropriate rituals, as well as for the exchange of tips and creation of rules on how to rear twins. For example, Funza, the twinship drum of the BaKongo, includes practical rules like, "if you give a gift or a bit of food to one twin, you must give the same gift to the other." "Do not strike twins, for they are holy children" (Ndibu, 1974, pp. 57-60).

Drums are significant as a concept across Bantu Africa because drums are the voice of ancestors or the spirit world. Often the drum represents the ancestor who was a member of the drum society in a previous generation and who is calling out, possessing, or identifying an individual among the living to join a particular drum. So a parent of twins will be told by the priest of the twin drum that "you are being nominated by such and such an ancestor and you must, therefore, join." This ideology of possession is academic in such cases as I have just mentioned (chiefship of the scrotal hernia and twinship) because possession is not at all apparent as a psychological phenomenon; it is simply that something occurs to a person and there, all of a sudden, is the affliction.

In some drums, the manifestation of psychic possession is more apparent. For example, the Tukuka drum of the southern Lunda peoples came into being in the 1940s and 1950s as a response of individuals experiencing nightmares about Europeans. That part of the world, today Zambia, was a British colony, and the response to intense interaction with whites in a colonial situation led frequently to people being haunted by the spirits of Europeans in dreams and nightmares (Turner, 1968).

Two further examples from Central African drums of affliction will suffice to illustrate the diversity of the institution. My favorite drum, Lemba, came into being in the seventeenth century and endured until the early twentieth century as a major public institution. It extended from the inland market at Mpumbu on Mulebo Pool, at the end of the thousand-mile-long inland river route of trade, to the coast. One could not go by river directly to the coast because of the rapids between the Mulebo Pool and the ocean, so the big market at the Pool channeled all the outgoing trade of ivory and slaves and the incoming trade of guns, cloth, and other European wares. Over the region from Mpumba market to the coast, north of the Zaire River, Lemba functioned as a ceremonial trading society to control the local markets and the trade routes, keeping them open and keeping the massive international trade from destroying society. In the mid-eighteenth century, annually 15,000 slaves were being shipped out of the three ports north of the Zaire River coast of Loango, Cabinda, and Malemba. These slaves were drawn from inland societies in which the chaotic impact was clearly perceived. The conflict of interest between economic reward and loss of the slaves may explain why Lemba's "governmental" function was channeled into the "drum of affliction" mold. It is an indication of the breadth and flexibility of Bantu African "medicine" that the redistributive ethic prevalent in these societies was imposed on the emerging mercantile elite. Merchants who became wealthy or powerful on the trade were perceived as, in some sense, "sick" or marginal. Lemba's medicine consisted of exorbitant fees and other civic duties, a good therapy — transformation anywhere for the profit motive (Janzen, 1979, 1982).

A final example of a Bantu drum of affliction comes from modern-day Kinshasa. There Zebola functions to bring together women lost in the big city: isolated single women; wives stuck at home whose husbands are away working or roaming around unproductively; and women adrift who need orientation, a fixed point in urban society (Corin, 1979). More will be offered on Zebola later in this chapter and on African "drums" as they relate to similar treating associations from other cultural traditions.

The gourd dance of the southern Plains Indian societies dates back to before the creation of reservations, when it was a warrior society among the Kiowa, Comanche, Cheyenne, and Arapaho. When the warriors put down their arms in the late nineteenth century and were placed on reservations in Oklahoma, the gourd dance served as a context to work out their frustrations, but the crisis that resulted from being forcefully put onto reservations was so terrible that the gourd dance died out; only the songs survived in the minds of some people. The peyote cult and the Native American Church followed in its place. At the end of the Vietnam war when all the veterans came home, again there were warriors who had turned in their guns. They were now sitting around in cities and towns in the southern Plains states not knowing what to do, drinking, often getting into trouble, and lacking a sense of orientation. The gourd dance reemerged as one such orientation, especially among Vietnam war veterans. Today, in the cities of the Plains states and on the reservations one finds active gourd chapters and clans. Gourd dances take place in the context of pow-wows and other public settings. There is an emphasis, in local chapters, on counseling and dancing together the unique pulsating circular gourd dance. Cheeves Coffey, Haskell Indian Junior College's student counselor, uses and participates in the gourd dance as the best treatment for an American Indian who has alcohol problems,* and this is widespread (Gephardt, 1977; Howard, 1976).

---

*Personal communications, 1978.

A leading Euroamerican "drum anonymous" again concerns alcohol – Alcoholics Anonymous (AA). Alcoholics Anonymous was brought into being in 1935 in Akron, Ohio, by an individual named Bill, whose public image remains anonymous. "Bill," a former alcoholic, contacted a friend who was still an alcoholic and persuaded him to stop drinking. The two of them contacted others, and so AA came into existence. Today it has a membership of at least 500,000, with 15,000 chapters in 40 countries and related organizations for spouses of alcoholics, Alanon, and for children, Alateen (AA, n.d.; Grainger, 1971).

Another anonymous help society of increasing national U.S. prominence, Parents Anonymous, was founded in Berkeley, California, in the late 1960s by, and for the purpose of helping, parents who abused their children. Parents Anonymous local chapters encourage former child abusers to refrain from beating their children and to help others abstain from this.

In passing, I must mention Synanon, a series of therapeutic communities for drug "addicts," founded on the model of AA, with the difference that they are residential units. Since the "rattlesnake incident" and Jonestown suicide-massacre in Guyana, Synanon's reputation has become that of a cultlike total institution. Numerous in-depth studies of Synanon's highly structured approach to drug rehabilitation have confirmed its effectiveness in many cases, however (Yablonsky, 1965).

To offset the association of drums anonymous groups with totalitarian cults, the emergence of this type of therapeutic maintenance model may be sketched in areas of physiological pathology but in which there are clear psychosocial overtones: coronary attack victims and subjects of organ transplants. There are hundreds of attempts to organize victims of heart attack into rehabilitation units in this country and elsewhere. I will focus on developments in post-coronary units in Germany, a society characterized by rationalist-bureaucratic, industrial norms. There the common victims of heart attack are middle-aged males who are successful, constructively aggressive, compulsively active, and generally at the prime of their life, at least in terms of their careers. When they have a heart attack they are suddenly crippled, psychologically and physically. Some of those many who survive the first attack become aware that they can no longer live the way they did and that the very nature of their life-style is what nearly destroyed them. Cardiac recovery and rehabilitation units, under the supervision of heart specialists, bring together victims and together they work on exercising and "slowing down." They continue to exercise together and to meet because they have found that they cannot come to terms with this transformation of character on their own. They can do it so much more easily if they have others around them in the same situation, sanctioning them to uphold the new life-style. And thus there emerges a permanent structure similar to the other organizations mentioned (Sonntag, 1978).*

Finally, I want to mention a yet unnamed type of anonymous society, found in the ad hoc attempts at contact on the part of organ donors and organ recipients and their next of kin. Efforts by the medical profession, for good legal reasons, to keep the organ donor-recipient relationship "anonymous" are repeatedly thwarted by an extraordinarily strong desire on the part of the recipient or the donor (and if deceased, their kin) to identify and get acquainted with the other side of the biological relationship created by the passage of the organ from the body of one person to another. Despite all the legal blocks often set up, it seems that in many cases they are successful in identifying the source or the final outcome of the organ and then in establishing a social relationship that continues for the duration of the lives involved. There is a need to come to terms with the existential problem of having a strange organ in their body (Fox and Swazey, 1978).

CHARACTERISTICS OF DRUMS ANONYMOUS

The drums anonymous briefly detailed in the foregoing paragraphs have a number of common characteristics, or close resemblances, that bear further scrutiny. The first of these concerns *recruitment*. This may take the form of a natural occurrence of a disease or misfortune; it may take the form of possession. It can take the form of a kind of election by those in it. Often the election process is self-selecting in that an individual's very behavior provides eligibility for membership in a group; this is true of twinship, or dreaming of Europeans, or finding oneself a returned Vietnam veteran without a job and not knowing what to do. Common to all is the feature

---

*William Arkinstall, personal communications, 1978.

that the new status making one eligible for belonging comes on the individual rather suddenly and in an overwhelming way, without the person being able to do anything about it.

The final eligibility for recruitment is the self-realization that the individual can do nothing about the problem. There is an overwhelming desire for help.

Yet, despite this initial helplessness, a further key characteristic of these groups is that once the initiation therapy process has begun, the "sufferer" gradually is transformed into a *healer*. In this characteristic, drums anonymous institutions offer a striking contrast to orthodox professional medical models. In the process that makes the sufferer into a healer, the affliction, the ill, or the evil is somehow converted into a virtue, an intriguing psychological and social process. Its particular cultural modes need further examination. In Central Africa, possession by an ancestor legitimates the illness as a virtue. It ennobles suffering; it gives the sufferer an identity; it helps name and situate the problem; and it suggests what the process has become, or must become. A Lemba song precisely identifies the process in these terms: "that which is the 'stab in the side' – the physical affliction – has become the path to the priesthood." The affliction is converted into a calling, suggesting the way in which the sufferer will be rehabilitated or emancipated and brought out of isolation into the midst of fellow sufferers turned healer. This feature is present across the gamut of drums anonymous under consideration.

As universal as the sufferer-to-healer characteristic may be, each drum anonymous has a precise *therapeutic mode* for its unique affliction. In the chiefship of scrotal hernia the "therapy" consists of re-creating the individual into a judge, thus providing a meaningful alternative role in society. In twinship the mode of therapy, once the shock of twins is absorbed, is that of learning the techniques of effective parenting and of coming to terms with one's superchildren or spirit children (i.e., twins). In Tukuka, the mode of therapy is to identify and expose the afflicting Europeans' spirit and thus to neutralize or to exorcise it. In Zebola, the Kinshasa women's drum, the mode of therapy is to fête the person being initiated in a large gathering, thereby making this isolated woman who is perhaps sorry for herself into a "Queen for a Day" in her coming out ceremony in Zebola, after which she has a fixed goal within Zebola. In Lemba the therapeutic mode consisted of making the men with profit motives pay exorbitant sums in the initiation fee. At the turn of the century in one area of Lower Zaire the fee was 25 pigs, several baskets of raffia cloth money, and the provision of a banquet for all of Lemba's members and all local inhabitants. A heavy dose of redistribution of goods was held to be excellent therapy for one who tended to cling to one's possessions. Also the Lemba neophyte with his major wife would go through a Lemba marriage, a highly sacred affair. Great emphasis in the Lemba marriage was placed on the maintenance of linkages of peace between localized communities and of support for the market network and the trade routes. Thus a type of marriage and gift redistribution were the "therapeutic" modes. In the gourd dance, sobriety is an important element in therapy, but it is coupled with mental purification and contemplation. Although the gourd dance is not acknowledged to be a religion, it has a strong element of asceticism to it, in the model of the sufferer turning healer. In some of the anonymous societies in the Euroamerican tradition, the therapeutic mode may take on the form of a type of conversion experience, or at least the conviction or acknowledgement on the part of candidates that they indeed need help. Alcoholics Anonymous has its 12 steps of membership, making explicit the acknowledgement of help. You must acknowledge, for example, that you have harmed others, you must identify them, and you must go to these people and straighten out the problems.

Despite the clearly religious elements of possession, asceticism, and conversion, most of the drums anonymous under discussion are *nonsectarian* in that one can belong to several at once. For example, a chief of the scrotal hernia was still a member of his village and his family. This membership in no way restricted his social life. Membership in drums of twinship is similar. Turner suggests that among the Ndembu a normal adult would belong to four or five drums for life. Now the question of whether they may become sectarian depends on the degree of their corporateness, a notion that derives from a particular tradition in social theory.

DRUMS AS CORPORATE INSTITUTIONS

I find it useful to hold up to drums anonymous the set of criteria that determines whether they are merely a corporate "category" of people, loosely affiliated because of their common characteristics, or whether they are a corporate "group" with common affairs, meetings, defined membership, an internal administrative structure and a conscious awareness of their organization vis-à-vis comparable organizations with which they may compete (Maine, 1960; Smith, 1974). Tukuka, the drum directed to those who had dreamed of Europeans, apparently never really made it to the status of corporate drum of affliction. There were no active local chapters; it was merely recognized that there were many people in the common category of this type of affliction who could have gotten organized into a drum. There was a small flourish of activity of a drumlike nature, but it fizzled out and then there were left people who had haunting dreams of Europeans without much to do about it. On the other hand, Lemba was an enormously influential drum and, although it was not centralized, it functionally substituted for a centralized kingdom. It even had a taxation system. In effect, it maintained the peace, it took care of the economy, and it was a type of welfare network. Its strong corporate fabric lasted three centuries.

It is thus conceivable that a drum anonymous could go through a process of fuller and fuller corporate group functioning and become a total institution, to be used for social control and co-optation. Lemba, for example, absorbed Pfemba, another drum that functioned as a midwife's organization and had to do with female fertility. Lemba, because it also was interested in the relationship between men and women and the marriages that tied together local communities, saw fit in the west to absorb Pfemba's medicines into its own medicine basket. There is the potential here then of these units becoming like centralized hierarchized medical establishments. At the other end of a continuum amorphous loosely linked categories of people will obtain.

This ebbing and flowing character of drums anonymous structure relates to another issue, namely the taxonomic focus it will assume within the general disease or problem taxonomy of the society. Briefly, it is apparent that these drums anonymous emerge in areas requiring permanent restructuring and maintenance, not of individuals beset with diseases or problems that merit a one-time solution but with those suffering chronic affliction. The sufferer never fully loses the illness. The affliction is seen as a permanent calling. For example, in Alcoholics Anonymous the members go through the ritual where they acknowledge that "once an alcoholic, always an alcoholic" and they will never forget this and they cannot forget it; it is inherent in them. So, too, heart attack victims in cardiac rehabilitation units know that they have had an attack or attacks, that they have this proclivity, and that it is inherent in them, a part of their history that they cannot eliminate.

STIGMA, SOCIAL CONTROL, AND MEDICALIZATION

The foregoing might raise the question of stigma and social control, of whether all these drums anonymous are not in reality methods by which a society medicalizes its culture in order to coerce people. If there really is no full cure in drums anonymous, but rather a permanent maintenance of the sick role at a kind of rehabilitative level, is not this truly a sophisticated version of medicalization for social and political control? Does it differ from instances in modern societies, in which dissidents have been declared psychiatrically deranged, giving the government license to permanently monitor them because they might ostensibly get out of control?

Well, some drums anonymous are conservative and others are revolutionary. Whether they are the one or the other depends on how, or if, they play into the hands of an even more centralized institution or act as a fairly autonomous social entity. I can see how anonymous associations could play into the hands of a powerful medical profession and become an extension of it. But if they steer clear of subordinate organizational involvement with more powerful organizations, then their function might be that of a critical independent body within the society, acting as a source of change. The gourd dance seems to lean in this direction. One of its key values is to make the young Plains man or woman who has had problems of identity or other problems into a more forceful, independent person. The gourd dance may be considered a network linking informally to the more militant American Indian Movement. On the other hand, it links informally to more conservative establishments in Midwestern society.

There is an example from Central Africa of a drum of affliction that existed in the Kingdom of Ruanda in the late nineteenth and early twentieth centuries. The kingdom was highly stratified into an elite royal clan and other noble and commoner castes. The Kubandwa drum was by contrast extremely egalitarian; in effect,

it recruited people suffering from conflicts of exclusion and strat-
ification into one common social bond, thus putting the drum
of affliction into the role of a revolutionary force within the
society.

THE ECONOMICS OF DRUMS ANONYMOUS

A final characteristic must be examined, namely the economic
dimension of drums anonymous. I have to deal with this because
medical planners or public policy makers may believe they have
learned of an institutional type that would alleviate the financial
burden of caring for all chronic cases and that we may now forget
about hospitals and asylums. That is not what is being said. If social
cost and manpower analyses are made of these institutions, it
becomes apparent that they require and consume a great deal of
human time. They represent an investment of time perhaps more
than of capital, but time may be translated to work, and work
translated to capital. So, what do they cost in terms of human time?
The Plains Indians convert sizeable portions of their hard-earned
wages and other cash incomes into ceremonial goods, such as
blankets, shawls, and even horses in some cases. In Plains Indian
society in general, and in the gourd dance in particular, these ceremonial goods are circulated in the mechanism of the "giveaway."
An individual who has recovered from a trauma, or experienced a
transition, or whose child has just been renamed, will distribute
large numbers of blankets, shawls, and other goods. Giveaways
represent an investment into the social network that constitutes the
gourd dance and beyond it the entire society of Plains Indians.
Thus, drums anonymous maintain social networks either on a limited
basis among their adherents, or they set up and extend supportive
networks throughout the society. Some, such as Lemba, "cost"
neophytes dearly in the creation of a mercantile elite; other cannot so visibly be seen to convert wealth to relations. But in the
Euroamerican anonymous groups, the periodic meetings and stay-
ing in touch and the telephoning are a great expenditure of time.
And that is what these units are all about — the creation of relationships and the maintenance of people in new or specially adapted
roles.

DRUMS ANONYMOUS: ACKNOWLEDGMENT
MADE OF HEALING

The type of therapeutic maintenance unit I have here called drums anonymous represents, I believe, a very widespread, if not universal and elemental mode of healing. The examples from the Euroamerican tradition (e.g., Alcoholics Anonymous, Parents Anonymous, cardiac rehabilitation units) suggest that it is a viable specific form of therapy for chronic afflictions of diffuse and multiple causation from physical, social, and psychological realms, with many other applications than have been mentioned. It is a model of care that stands midway, organizationally, between high-cost specialist's care of the dependent single patient and the totally aprofessional practice of folk medicine.

REFERENCES

Alcoholics Anonymous. n.d. *44 Questions*. New York.

Corin, E. 1979. A Possession Psychotherapy in an Urban Setting: Zebola in Kinshasa. In *The Social History of Disease and Medicine in Africa*, ed. J. M. Janzen and S. Feierman. Oxford: Pergamon. Special Issue *Soc. Sci. Med.* 13B(4).

De Sousberghe, L. 1958. *L'Art Pende*. Brussels: L'Académie Royale des Sciences Coloniales (Tome IX, fasc. 2 Beaux-Arts).

Fox, R., and Swazey, J. 1978. *The Courage to Fail: A Social View of Organ Transplants and Dialysis*. Chicago: University of Chicago Press.

Gephardt, L. 1977. *The Affective Structure of the Gourd Dance*, Anthropology M.A. thesis. Lawrence: University of Kansas.

Grainger, D. 1971. Fieldnotes on Alcoholics Anonymous. Montreal (unpublished notes).

Howard, J. H. 1976. The Plains Gourd Dance as a Revitalization Movement. *Am. Ethnologist* 2:243-59.

Janzen, J. 1979. Ideologies and Institutions in the Precolonial History of Equatorial African Therapeutic Systems. In *The Social History of Disease and Medicine in Africa*, ed. J. M. Janzen and S. Feierman, pp. 317-26. Oxford: Pergamon.

———. 1982. *Lemba 1650-1930: A Drum of Affliction in Africa and the New World*. New York: Garland.

Maine, H. 1960. *Ancient Law*. London: Dent.

Ndibu, J. 1974. Father of Twins. In *An Anthology of Kongo Religion*, ed. J. M. Janzen and W. MacGaffey, pp. 57-59. Lawrence: University of Kansas Publications in Anthropology 5.

Smith, M. G. 1974. *Corporations and Society*. London: Duckworth.

Sonntag, W. 1978. "Nach dem Herzinfarkt." *Die Zeit*, 26 (30 June).
Turner, V. W. 1968. *Drums of Affliction*. Oxford: Clarendon.
_____ . 1969. *The Ritual Process*. Chicago: Aldine.
Yablonsky, L. 1965. *Synanon: The Tunnel Back*. Baltimore: Penguin Books.

11

COMMUNAL DECISION MAKING:
A Demedicalization Model from the Yugoslavian Health Care System

Robert L. Berg

The evolution of national health programs in countries or jurisdictions that have had strong but diverse tribal or communal organizations and expectations presents cultural confrontations in regard to both administrative mechanisms and technological choices.

In Yugoslavia, health care developments in the past 30 years have been principally concerned with administrative mechanism. There is considerable folk medicine practiced, especially among older people in rural areas where medical facilities may be remote. In former Turkish territories much of this is based on Moslem traditions. However, these are fading practices. This chapter focuses on the administrative mechanisms that have been devised to deal with resource allocation in a diverse country with regions of intense nationalism and communal pride (Berg, Brooks, and Savicevic, 1976).

Yugoslavia has responded to local nationalism by assigning to each republic the major administrative responsibilities for the activities of government. Furthermore, within each republic (the smallest, Montenegro, has only 400,000 inhabitants), health care planning is largely left to communal associations averaging 200,000 inhabitants. A further accommodation to parochial concerns has been set up. Within each communal association a separate health insurance plan exists for farmers, as compared with other workers. Furthermore, special arrangements are provided for independent workers such as artists, musicians, and small private entrepreneurs. The decision to allow so much local option was a product of the intense individualism of Yugoslav peasants, especially in mountainous regions with poor transport. In these areas, although the standard of living is low, there is such intense feeling against large cooperative organizations that only minor efforts have been directed toward communal farming, for example.

The characteristic health care organization at the communal association unit level involves a set of independent providers on the one hand and an insurance scheme on the other. These are very similar to the Blue Cross organizations in the United States. Independent provider groups such as hospitals, ambulatory clinics, emergency services, and drug stores are each independent enterprises. Internal decisions are made democratically, and each functions quite separately from the other components of the health care system. The social insurance organization is a service organization that functions to distribute funds and monitor their use by the providers. Their role in collecting the funds is minimal, since each communal association decides what total monies will be collected each year on the basis of payroll tax for a wide variety of health, education, and welfare programs. Thus, each year the individual communal association has decided what will be spent for health and must then allocate this single pot of money to the various health care needs of the community.

The decision body is a special assembly. In the beginning this was made up entirely of consumer representatives. Over the past ten years it became evident that consumer understanding of the total workings of the health care system was faulty in some cases. As a result, the current arrangement allows for the assembly to include one-third providers and one-third elected government officials. Nevertheless, the feedback to the grass roots is intimate and direct. Each representative to the health assembly is elected from a general communal health assembly that is made up of direct representatives from every enterprise in the community. These individuals are responsible for explaining to their constituency why the money is spent as it is or to present to the assembly their arguments for larger allocations for given programs. Frequently, basic policy issues are taken back to the primary electorate for referenda.

How successful is this approach in bringing to the average citizen the sense of involvement and decision making? As in most multiple-tiered systems of decision making, most citizens feel remote from the ultimate decision but not powerless. The complaints about health care are roughly the same as in the United States: it costs too much and one waits too long. There are interesting options available to citizens, however. They may seek an illegal consultation with a physician outside office hours. This is widespread, and considerable physician income is generated thereby. They may reduce the waiting time by paying a tip to the physician involved either in the hospital or in the clinic. In fact, there is a widely known standard fee to pay one's general practitioner to get the referral slip to the hospital in time of need. Furthermore, there are well-established norms for tips to the personnel inside hospitals, including doctors, nurses, and aides. Without such tipping the care patients receive may be minimal.

Beyond these economic issues, the system is more responsive to local mores and expectations since the decisions are made at close hand and most consumers know personally either members of the insurance assembly or of the communal primary level assembly that elects them. Personal interference in favor of a colleague or friend is widespread in all Yugoslav institutions, and in the health system it functions much as in the United States. Unfortunately, there have been few controlled studies of whether satisfaction or patient compliance is substantially greater under such an arrangement than one with federal control.

The relationship of the Yugoslav health system to medicalization is worth noting. In a situation in which all health monies come from a single pool, it becomes painfully clear that there are too few resources to do all things for all people. There is, then, a strong disincentive to expand the arena of health care expenditures to marginal areas. Indeed, there is every reason to pull back from programs that might be picked up by the welfare or educational pockets of the communal budget.

The feature of the system that makes this operational is the availability of a single pool of money. Once allocated there can be no further income. Contingency funds may be set aside, but they will not be substantial given the tight competition for funds. At first glance the arrangement would seem to be limited to fixed salary arrangements and to rule out fee for service practice. In the case of hospitals, however, reimbursement is not necessarily limited to fixed budgets. Both per diem and case mix reimbursements have been explored. But as is the case with foundation plans in the United States in which doctors may submit fees to a fixed insurance pool, when the money runs low payments, may have to be prorated. Each part of the system, whether it be hospitals, clinics, emergency services, or pharmacies, may try to expand its domain. But the only opportunity to "medicalize" the welfare system, for example, would require the welfare agencies to give up some of their piece of pie. That expansion attempt would be out in the open, negotiated at the level of the communal association. There can be no creeping medicalization.

Dissatisfaction with the style of practice can lead to specified conditions before budgets are awarded. Cooperation with schools, with welfare agencies, or even with traditional healers might be required as part of the budgeted activities. Holistic health movements have not surfaced in Yugoslavia, but major emphasis has been placed on comprehensive primary care that is available even in remote areas.

Those concerned about medicalization in other countries might follow Yugoslavia's ingenious solution. In the United States there are programs and experiments in fixed budgeting for health care for defined populations. These include comprehensive care plans such as Kaiser-Permanente programs as well as fixed reimbursement experiments for hospitals. Such programs limit expenditures for defined populations, and they discourage expansion into new areas of health care, but they may inhibit desired expansion into such fields as preventive services. The dilemma is posed yet again: can cost containment and the avoidance of medicalization be overdone?

REFERENCE

Berg, R. L.; Brooks, M. R., Jr.; and Savicevic, M. 1976. Health Care in Yugoslavia and the United States. Fogarty International Center Proceedings No. 34, DHEW Publication No. (NIH) 75-911.

12

MEDICALIZATION AND METAPHOR:
Their Meanings in Culture

Lola Romanucci-Ross

Medicalization can be described as the structuring of the somatic drama through the interpretation of health and illness by the *providers* of health care imposed on the *consumers* of health care. Providers also perpetuate such structuring within their own sub-culture through codes of propriety in training, problem-recognition, and problem-solution in pathology and dysfunction. This structuring called "medicalization" is a cultural process, for culture can be described as the structuring and processing of information. As in the culmination of all social movements, the structure becomes "reified." A consensus today seems to indicate that there are many agreed-upon needed changes in the forum of medicalizers and medicalized.

I carried out field research in a "primitive" culture when it was possible to observe and record incipient inroads of medicalization among such groups. I noted a "hierarchy of resort of curative practices" (Schwartz, 1969) and demonstrated that a commonality exists in concepts of health and sickness in societies of a certain level of complexity (Landy, 1977).

Using the statistical and descriptive material collected in my own fieldwork and that available from the fieldnotes of Fortune (1935), Mead, (1930, 1956), and Schwartz (1962, 1963), I wrote about shifting "game" strategies in curing events, when the choices were multiple and reflected varying degrees of deculturation and acculturation. Priorities and sequentiality of selected curing procedures could be predicted. Disease causes were distinguishable through several categories, both impersonal and interpersonal.

Because the somatic drama is culturally informed, one must consider the illness-health continuum as grounded in the sensory perceptions of the world and how they are registered as knowledge configurations for further receiving (Bateson, 1979). How is consensus about health and illness arrived at from the syntactical to the rhetorical and from the "coding" on the many levels of organization of experience?

Here we will consider this view in our contemporary society: how does the study of a simple primitive group illuminate definitions of health and illness, and the processes of discovery, and classification of causality, the former being further discriminated into natural and supernatural and the latter into cursing or witchcraft from within the group or from an outside group. Inquiries leading to such categorical diagnostics were "nested" in shifting culture contact situations, and diagnoses varied accordingly. Depending on which coordinates one located the illness episode, a differing series of resort patterning in terms of first and follow-up strategies could be predictably found. In historical moments of high acculturation, Western medicine was the first choice, to be followed, in case of failure, by the more traditional modes, although if these also failed, reversion to Western medicine in another attempt was common.

More typical was a counteracculturative sequence. Here the primary treatment of herbs and hot leaf applications or ingested infusions was followed by therapy by the local healer. Then, the Aid Post Orderly (the local version of allopathic Western medicine) was used, followed by the hospital at the Australian Naval Base, as a last resort. Each choice had a separate sociomoral function.

In the recent present, it is noted that diagnoses and curing attempts of the first resort are counteracculturative.* After an epidemic of "sudden death" of men mostly in their 50s in 1978, victims are now described as having been struck down by the angry ghosts of the dead; even the terminology is pre-Western. Those who die by slowly wasting away are said to be victims of sorcery. In Pere Village those who are ill are once more imploring the skulls of

---

*Ted Schwartz, personal communication.

the dead fathers to ask them why they are the targets of so much paternal harshness and beg to be healed and made whole once more — as in the past (Fortune, 1935). While the living are digging up skulls to entreat and bones to carry home for divination purposes, the dead being implored are having committee meetings with Jesus, as they did during the cult revival period (Schwartz, 1962). This reshaped behavior follows a short period of political independence declared in the late 1960s for Papua New Guinea. In this period we see that Western medicine is being forced into a retrenchment that is heralded with a new distrust of hospitals and Western-trained physicians.

Facilitating the understanding of such occurrences must be the recognition that there is a coding to be deciphered in the metaphorical linkages of the "world view" (belief systems) or "knowledge configurations" (Foucault, 1969). By the time of the more recent writing on Melanesian medicine, metaphor had to be taken into account as well as rational structures of thought. I attempted to demonstrate with cultural specificity how what had been learned of perception and imagery affected configurations of knowledge in the same primitive culture previously analyzed for hierarchy of resort (Romanucci-Ross, 1979).

FROM PRIMITIVE TO FOLK MEDICINE

What can "folk medical practice" add to our total understanding of health care in complex societies? Any culture permits an illness to play various roles, such as asserting individual needs and eliciting certain kinds of behavior from others. *Illness is therefore a negotiable event.* So there are illnesses that can be ignored or that may be exaggerated. One who believes oneself to be ill will (usually) seek confirmation from others and only then begin the journey-cure. These features of illness are applicable in complex societies as well as in primitive and peasant cultures. Woods and Graves (1976) established a framework for the changing patterns of curative resort utilization in a rural community of Guatemala and, when quantifying socioeconomic variables and health-related behavior, found interesting correlations. Woods (1977) also looked for acculturative trends among Ladinos and Indians. These studies well demonstrate the transfer ability of certain basic concepts. In a rural village in Mexico studied over a long period (Romanucci-Ross, 1973; see also Fromm and Maccoby, 1970), I had noted that illness was the most common occasion for relating to others the trajectory of one's life experiences or for indicating aspirations and frustrations. How system balance is operant in the maintenance of health relates to much that is observed in primitive, peasant, or more complex cultural settings. People who do not use words such as "homeostasis" nevertheless have a notion of it.

For example, among a number of American Indians, illness is related to a temporary power imbalance. All things and people have inherent or acquired powers; illness is caused by an external power that overwhelms the power within the individual. In the curing process powers are invoked by the healer who understands which "balances" must be brought to bear. The healer will take care, for example, in preparing herbal decoctions to have the proper combination of "male" and "female" herbs.

Similarly, we find in Central and South America "hot" and "cold" categories in which food or other environmental stimuli are placed (see Foster, 1978). Any number of physical-disorder states from discomfort to serious illness are attributed to having eaten, drunk, or abided something too "hot" or too "cold." Descriptors of these extremes are puzzling because they do not coincide appropriately with temperatures, taste, or feel. But when regarded as another instance of the need to keep in balance the elements taken into the body or surrounding the body, it is a view that can "make sense." In contemporary California, we know that some immigrants did not abandon these concepts in Mexico as "hot" and "cold." Attributes are now attached by these immigrants to our consumer products; Coca-Cola is "hot" because its color approximates that of brown sugar, and Seven-Up is "cold" because of its resemblance to lime juice. We see that even though the particulars in the place of origin may not always be encountered in the new environment, the structure of the thought system and its rules for attribution continue, with new elements placed into categories for which they qualify. European immigrants to the United States have furnished many examples of this process.

TO THE COMPLEXITIES OF OPEN SOCIETIES

Folk practitioners have something to offer the traditional Western providers of health care who try to interpret symptom reporting and the range of responses to their diagnoses and prescriptions. Use of folk practitioners as mediators has worked among the Navaho (Adair and Deuschle, 1970). The model could be followed with profit in urban centers of the United States. Puerto Ricans in American cities refer to personal, natural causes as well as supernatural causes of disease and illness. Delgado (1979) emphasizes that their healers have specialized knowledge. One finds the *espiritista* or medium, the *santero* or metaphysical healer for personalistic etiologies of illness, the *santiquador* for the laying-on-of-hands, and the herbalist for "natural" illnesses. Delgado emphasizes that members of the Puerto Rican community will most often seek treatment that is "culturally specific and culturally based because their expectations clash with a health care system that is not equipped to deal with some of these expectations" (Delgado, 1979, p. 788). Such researches could aid communication between consumers and providers of health care. Like others who suggest how this should come about, Delgado places all the burden of learning and ministering learned lessons on the providers. His conclusions have the advantage of high agreement with conclusions and recommendations of other studies in medical anthropology. Such unilateral efforts by providers, however, have not occurred with the force required to make a significant difference in health care delivery nor is this likely to happen in a sustained manner. We have more than sufficient evidence to assert that positive attitudes emerge and multiply between parties who engage in exchanges that are mutually rewarding (Byrne and Rhamey, 1965; Lott and Lott, 1969).

Even among Americans who are not considered minorities there is a hierarchy of resort in curative practices, as Wallis and Morley (1976) indicate. They look at populations who consult chiropractors, osteopaths, and others who claim the supremacy of their assumptions about healing. At the very least they feel that although they may not be acceptable to conventional medical practitioners they could be complementary to their efforts by being included in the referral system. Claims to legitimacy in authoritativeness in medicine represent a long struggle in our society, particularly that between allopathic medicine and osteopathy. Cohen (1980) documents the struggle that she interprets as the ascendancy of one social movement over another. Until the beginning of this century, the allopathic physician was not held in the highest esteem by much of the voting and articulate public. Allopathic medicine was, and to some extent still is, based on the principles of opposites; the goal is to bring the system back into balance, much like the "hot" and "cold" view. Illness was also viewed by this school as being caused by external agents. Homeopathy, in contrast, worked with similarities rather than differences; one ingested very small doses of what one "had" to restore system balance in the belief that "like cures like" (Inglis, 1964). Osteopathy, introduced after 1860 by Andrew Taylor Still, maintained that pharmaceutical drugs were toxic agents, that the body should be viewed as a whole and within its econiche, and that cure would be found by realigning the structure of the body by manipulation. The allopaths carried the field through concerted action (i.e., professional societies, professional journals, the 1910 Flexner Report with its declaration and definition of orthodox medical scientism). Through such actions they pushed for standards of medical practice and for abhorrence of quacks (all who were not allopaths), and they carried a social movement to political victory (Fletcher and Fletcher, 1979; Wilson, 1979). It should not be left unmentioned that the victorious group did indeed borrow concepts that made "scientific sense" from the marginal medicine men and did, if not as quickly as some patients and their families might have wished, drop some of their own practices that were ineffective, detrimental, or lethal to their patients, such as bloodletting for yellow fever (see Rush, 1794). We have the historical time span in our own culture to survey and examine medical practice strategies to learn about hierarchies of resort of curing and healing by our own professionals as they jockeyed for ascendancy and control.

DEATH'S BODY

The training process of the physician and other health professionals sets them apart from the vast majority of their patients who have differing inflections of the shared basic common culture. Members of these groups have their differences in the understanding of "person" and may differ from the conventional medical view that what is meant by illness is error introduced into the (psychosomatic) system. All recognize system error. But communication beyond that leaves much to be desired, as patients vacillate along a credulity continuum (along with primitives and peasants). Whatever the doctor's choices, medicalization is the enculturation process that begins this discourse about illness and this medical "reality."

Consider the example of the corpse in the late eighteenth and early nineteenth centuries. Anti-intellectual and antiscientific attitudes in the general public imposed a context of learning medicine from a corpse, acquired in colleagueship with "body snatchers." Cohen's study (1980) documents that these practices of physicians and their professors were seen by the public up to the middle part of the nineteenth century as sacreligious, perverted, and absurd. Dissection and "grave robbing" were viewed with an especial horror. The doctors who studied and did research with such materials saw their public detractors as short-sighted, uneducated, and superstitious. Dissection riots occurred in Philadelphia and Baltimore (see Marks and Beatty, 1973; Shafer, 1936). It is rather that the manner of learning had to have an effect on the medical student who viewed himself and the body under study as a quite different object. The student learned to relate the corpse to the solving of problems and so learned in terms of static and momentary cause and effect relationships. This produces a cross-sectional rather than a longitudinal problem-solving orientation.

The ethos and mystique of a profession grows out of the transformed shadows of its cultural survivals. Body snatching took place at night to avoid lynching by an angry public. The corpse then had to be dismembered so that it would not be recognized. Corpses are passive and they are not colleagues, so that the expectation is that the patient will assume the same attributes. Whatever is learned from the corpse has to be learned anew from the living body, but the *affect* and the *context* of the original lessons are not wiped out.

INFORMATION DISSEMINATION

Medicalization as the structuring of information on health and illness may emanate principally *but not exclusively* from the providers of health care. Indeed, with even greater force and more lasting effects it comes from advertising and the professions' "throw-away" journals from which the practitioner gets much of the current information. The advertising world is a repository of all techniques of persuasion; the consumer is assailed with juxtapositions of medications of dietary supplements with powerful symbols of attractiveness such as sexuality and wealth. One survey showed that 80 percent of health-related ads were false or misleading (Fromm and Maccoby,

1970) and also revealed that these misconceptions were believed to be accurate. Hovland and Weiss (1951) showed that after four weeks the knowledge of source of information (classified as one of high or one of low credibility) disappeared almost completely in the subjects. What remained was the message concerning, in this case, whether histamines should or should not continue to be sold without prescription by a physician.

Festinger (1957) held that when two "cognitions" that are in conflict are held at the same time, an individual or group is motivated to abolish or weaken the dissonance. I think it can be shown that this does not always apply in the doctor-patient relationship. Quite the contrary seemed to obtain in researches on religious cult behavior in Melanesia (Schwartz, 1963), where dissonant interpretations of events only fortified the need for even stronger devoted believing in the supernatural occurrences that were to happen and a more total investment in the belief that these occurrences were absolutely going to take place. In Melanesia (Manus), when material goods from the departed ancestors did not appear after proper ritual disposal of native-style properties, belief in the cult was strengthened. In doubt was the total commitment of the believers who were exhorted only to believe more completely and invest more totally in showing their belief in the outcome. So, too, was this noted in the cases of medical events I was studying. Failure of cure did not occasion an examination of the assumptions of native categories. Failure of cure, however, did reinforce beliefs that Western medicine did not cure really serious illness, that which occurred because of place, because of kinship, or because of witchcraft (Schwartz, 1969). In our culture, a patient will seek out a doctor at no small cost but then will not follow the advice that was given: consider the case of the smoker.

The parameters of quality assessment are many, and outcomes may or may not be related to following advice that comes from conventional medical sources. We know that compliance is not a reliable covariant of a felicitous outcome. Most information about health matters, as indicated above, comes through the journalistic medium to both the patient population and the health care providers. As such, it is subject to the style of journalism with its leads and cut-off points, its juxtaposed tableaux with a superimposed message of its own. Information from the Food and Drug Administration (FDA) or other government sources tends to be ignored (as on the hazards of smoking) or bitterly fought by vested interests (as on carcinogens in food additives, air, and water).

However, attitudinal changes do come about in ways that may surprise some of us. A dentist I know conducted his own investigation over a period of years. He found that to tell a woman that her gums and teeth may be damaged by smoking presents a much greater likelihood that she will give up the habit than telling her cigarette smoking may cause cancer or heart disease.

SOME CONCLUSIONS

Culture is the structuring and processing of information, but it is also all the residues that in time accumulate and influence indirectly the structuring and the processing. It would be well to develop a method to look at how imagery and perception interlace to exercise the selectivity and stylizing effects on the generated knowledge configurations (Romanucci-Ross, 1979). But for the present, we can at least postulate transactions and exchange within a social relations context. Emerson (1962, 1976), a social exchange theorist, maintains that there is reciprocity in the experimentor and the "experimentee" relation. We would add the concept that there is a stream-of-consciousness in each exchanging party. The consciousness continuums allow for points of real communication. It also allows for many points of mismatch of codes and messages. The physician has a body of information constantly, if minimally, transformed while going from patient to patient and interprets this information cross-sectionally. The patient has a longitudinal experiential history of an illness as it is presenting and a personal calculus of mishaps, misfortunes, and optimization strategies for resolution of the problem.

Within our problem orientation, medicalization can be viewed, as indeed it is by many, as attempts by power holders to leave the dependent patient little choice that the individual would find acceptable. Because of the too often *ignored consciousness of process*, this state of affairs has occasioned attempts that constitute islands of collusion between some patients and marginal healers to begin counteracculturative movements in medical care. It is to be hoped that conventional allopathic medicine, will, as it has in the past, assimilate what is scientifically valid into its own corpus of knowledge and, at the same time, broaden its hypotheses about health and behavior in the cultural context. We share with cultural groups of less complexity and less internal diversity the shifting game strategies of confronting illness to regain health. We may be on opposite ends of the medicalization continuum, but we all negotiate health care and identity seeking to retain the option of alternativity in seeking remedies to unhappy physical and mental states of disorder. We all seek a formula for colleagueship with our health care providers.

REFERENCES

Adair, J., and Deuschle, K. 1970. *The People's Health: Anthropology and Medicine in a Navaho Community*. New York: Appleton-Century-Crofts.

Bateson, G. 1979. *Mind and Nature: A Necessary Unity*. New York: Dutton.

Byrne, D., and Rhamey, R. 1965. Magnitude of Reinforcement as a Determinant of Attraction. *J. Personal Soc. Psychol.* 2:889-99.

Cohen, M. 1980. Medical Social Movements in the United States 1830-1979: The Case of Osteopathy. Ph.D. dissertation, University of California, San Diego, La Jolla.

Delgado, M. 1979. Puerto Rican Healers in the Big Cities. *Forum on Medicine* Vol. II, pp. 784-93.

Emerson, R. M. 1962. Power-Dependence Relations. *Am. Soc. Rev.* 27(1):31-41.

———. 1976. Social Exchange Theory. *Ann. Rev. Sociol.* 2:335-52.

Festinger, L. 1957. *A Theory of Cognitive Dissonance*. Evanston, Ill.: Row, Peterson.

Fletcher, R. H., and Fletcher, S. W. 1979. Clinical Research in General Medical Journals: A 30-year Perspective. *N. Eng. J. Med.* 301:180-83.

Flexner, A. 1972. *Medical Education in the United States and Canada — A Report to the Carnegie Foundation for the Advancement of Teaching*. New York: Arno Press (reprint of 1910 book).

Fortune, R. F. 1935. *Manus Religion*. Philadelphia: American Philosophical Society.

Foster, G., and Anderson, B. G. 1978. *Medical Anthropology*. New York: John Wiley & Sons.

Foucault, M. 1969. *L'Archaeologie du Savoir*. Paris: Gallimard.

Fromm, E., and Maccoby, M. 1970. *Social Character in a Mexican Village*. Englewood Cliffs, N.J.: Prentice-Hall.

Hovland, C. I., and Weiss, W. 1951. The Influence of Source Credibility on Communication Effectiveness. *Public Opinion Q.* 15:635-50.

Inglis, B. 1964. *The Case for Unorthodox Medicine*. New York: Putnam.

Landy, D. 1977. *Culture, Disease and Healing: Studies in Medical Anthropology*. New York: Macmillan.

Lott, B., and Lott, J. 1969. Liked and Disliked Persons as Reinforcing Stimuli. *J. Personal Soc. Res.* 11:129-37.

Marks, G., and Beatty, W. K. 1973. *The Story of Medicine in America.* New York: Scribner.

Mead, M. 1930. *Growing up in New Guinea.* New York: Morrow.

———. 1956. *New Lives for Old: Cultural Transformation Manus 1928-1953.* New York: Morrow.

Nelson, R. B., III. 1979. Are Clinical Trials Pseudoscience? *Forum on Medicine* Vol. II.

Romanucci-Ross, L. 1973. *Conflict, Violence and Morality in a Mexican Village.* Palo Alto, Calif.: Mayfield Publishing Company.

———. 1979. Melanesian Medicine: Beyond Culture to Method. In *Culture and Curing: Anthropological Perspectives on Traditional Medical Beliefs and Practices,* ed. P. Morley and R. Wallis. Pittsburgh: University of Pittsburgh Press (1978 London: Peter Owens Ltd.).

Rush, B. 1794. *An Account of the Bilious Remitting Yellow Fever as it Appeared in the City of Philadelphia 1793.* Philadelphia: T. Dobson.

Shafer, H. B. 1936. *The American Medical Profession 1783 to 1850.* New York: AMS Press.

Schwartz, L. R. 1969. The Hierarchy of Resort in Curative Practices: The Admiralty Islands, Melanesia. *J. Health Soc. Behavior* 10:201-9.

Schwartz, T. 1962. *The Paliau Movement in the Admiralty Islands 1946-1954.* New York: Anthropological Papers of the American Museum of Natural History vol. 49, part 2.

———. 1963. Systems of Areal Integration: Some Considerations Based on the Admiralty Islands of Northern Melanesia. *Anthropol. Forum* 1(1):56-97.

Wallis, R., and Morley, P., eds. 1976. *Marginal Medicine.* New York: Free Press.

Woods, C. 1977. Alternative Curing Strategies in a Changing Medical Situation. *Med. Anthropol.* 3(1):25-54.

Woods, C., and Graves, T. 1976. The Process of Medical Change in a Highland Guatemalan Town. In *Medical Anthropology,* ed. F. X. Grolling. The Hague: Mouton.

13

MEDICALIZATION AND PHYSICIAN SOCIALIZATION

John-Henry Pfifferling

OVERVIEW

Medicalization is an accretionary process associated with professional training in American medicine. Trainees learn to filter "relevant" data through a screen that is ruled by a set of images that are derived from a medically ethnocentric world view. These images are most highly valued, and nonmedical factors are discounted. The trainees internalize this model, out-of-their awareness, until they are confronted by an alternative world view, such as, "my feelings are not being addressed, only my organs, Doctor." It is my thesis that the medicalized view distorts physician's value systems and may harm both the physician (and the physician's family) and the patient. These models may oppose behavior that is in the patient's and the physician's best interest since they reinforce dependency by the patient on a medical gatekeeping system and they pressure the physician to be more responsible than necessary in many patient-doctor encounters.

This chapter focuses on identifying some medicalized values that permeate the medical culture and suggest how they might contribute to segmented and often uncoordinated medical care. The socialization or professionalization process and its resulting limiting world view will be considered as one cause of faulty patient-doctor, doctor-doctor, and doctor-health worker communication.

MEDICAL SOCIALIZATION

The process of the social and professional molding of an individual into a physician has been labeled "medical socialization." A body of literature concerned with this process has been produced by medical educators, sociologists, psychologists, and, more recently, psychiatrists. As would be expected, these different disciplines have stressed different themes in describing medical socialization. Sociologists have been primarily interested in student cultures as adaptive responses to a particular institutional setting. They have stressed the mediating role that student culture has played in responding to different profession-perceived enculturating functions, the various structural differences in different schools, and the molding image of the student-physician. Psychological studies have dealt with personality differences among students and the association between these differences and future medical practice decisions, especially the choice of specialties.

Woven throughout these studies is a prototypical orientation toward medicine as *the* profession. The medical profession assumes that a preprofessional aspires to gain a self-image that reflects control of the content, clients, organization, and self-regulation of medical professional responsibilities. It is assumed by most physicians in training that ultimately their profession will be autonomous in their workplace, training of future physicians, regulation of medical quality, and in defining "medical work." Official and public sanctions and mandates support the special place that the medical profession enjoys in contemporary occupations.

Current policy regarding the mandated autonomy of the medical profession is rethinking to a dramatic extent the control by the medical profession of quality assessment. This means that physician leadership and control of health decision-making actions will be challenged to a greater degree than expected by physicians. Currently, many assumptions are being considered as myths that fuel unrealistic expectations.

Just as current federal policy is rethinking its massive financial role in supporting the medical-health establishment and places the burden of proof on those who would provide more and costlier services, so are consumers rethinking their dependency on physicians as sole custodians of costly medical labels.

Extreme social statements describe American society as medicalized to such an extent that medical gatekeepers have triumphed over individual autonomy (Fox, 1977; Illich, 1976). It is alleged that American society has not only become medicalized but that it has become overmedicalized. Demedicalization as a phenomenon will come to pass, according to Illich's supporters, who sacramentally celebrate the freedom and the healing power of the individual.

THE MEDICALIZATION CRITIQUE

Medicalization from the critic's view refers to the inordinate dependence of the individual on the medical establishment. The establishment has become a threat to health. The case has been made by Illich et al. that the current medical care system (both in the United States and as exported internationally) if left to its personnel, incremental, and technological growth will act as a cancer on the American people. These critics posit that more people will contract disease produced by being exposed to hospital infections and other risks only encountered in medical-associated settings than those needing to enter the hospital. More people will have drug-induced reactions than there are drug types. The combination of effects produced by polydrug interactions and physician-generated iatrogenic interactions will produce new and uncontrollable diseases.

Medicalization also refers to the progressive usurping by professionalized medicine of domains that were traditionally the responsibility of friends, family, employers, the ministry, and other support populations. Health has left the spiritual and personal domain and become a medically controlled territory. Most recently there has been a continuing divestment of categories away from crime, morality, and deviancy toward disease as an explanatory framework: nonillness has become illness. Compulsive drinking, eating, smoking, and sexuality have all entered the physician's content realm. As Fox (1977) has written:

> if we include into what is considered sickness or, at least, non-health in the United States, disorders manifested by subjective symptoms which are not brought to the medical profession for diagnosis and treatment, but which do not differ significantly from those that are, then almost everyone in the society can be regarded as in some way "sick." (p. 11)

Taken to its extreme, if the medical profession becomes institutionally in control of prevention and the labels of risk associated with prevention, then the healthy individual becomes a rarity. Almost everyone has some form of subclinical disease, or potential disease, and those that monitor individual risk statuses will have powerful labeling tools at their control. Incurable illness may be diagnosed earlier, and "cardiac cripples" will multiply. With uncontrolled use of early diagnostic screening tests (with questionable yields), the potential for mislabeling, bias, error, and iatrogenic harm may increase dramatically.

Assuming that this global expansion of health "territory" continues unabated we can medicalize everyone. But medicalization also produces a counter trend: activated individuals who wish to divest themselves of dependency and to prevent personal medical co-optation. The self-care movement has not only become a fashionable phenomenon, but it has recruited significant numbers of medical professionals into its ranks. Alternative healing strategies easily become adapted by self-care groups, who do not have faith in slow, scientific validation.

Medical professionals themselves resent the technological displacement of their healing power by superspecialized technology and technologists. As physicians become more technologically dependent for their healing success, they progressively lose their own revitalizing from the human bonding associated with being a doctor. As physicians become less secure, their dormant but intimate ally resurfaces in a new guise: patient participation. The triumph of medical elitism inexorably leads to the alienation of an inviolable bond: doctors and patients. It is my opinion that this symbiotic partnership can not be severed for long without regenerating.

PERSONAL MEDICALIZATION

The ritual process of medical education is demanding. The physician in training not only acquires familiarity with telescoped information but also internalizes physician-role attitudes and values. Developmentally this person must accommodate to a decreased allowance for idealism, a denial of the clinical role of empathy in problem-solving, a permanent tolerance of uncertainty, and a perfectionistic quest for status.

Becker et al. (1961) and Miller (1970) have shown that adjustment to the physician role requires a continual reduction of the social and personal continuity of peer support. As they progress medical students also must readjust cognitive standards. The academic gamesmanship of the preclinical years is very different from roundsmanship in the clinical and house staff years.

The process of becoming a medical school graduate prepares one for denial: denial of personal affect, denial of the patient's own "clinical" construction of reality, denial of empathy, and denial of illness as a creative teacher. As one masters a spiraling body of information, one learns to deny metaphorical intuitions and the gut wisdom of the generalist. Mastery closes as well as opens, overpowers as well as inflates, and in modern medicine culminates in the prestige of specialty status. Biomedical disease is a tantalizing monster that demands the ritual sacrifice of humanism, idealism, two-way communication, and the human drive toward flexible curiosity.

As medical students and house staff become socialized to a more limited world view (a medicocentric vision), they gain status and cognitive assets. But what do they lose? They lose (1) their healing vision, (2) their respect for the creative teaching implicit in coping with illness, (3) their partnership with support persons and support resources (modern medical territorial issues deride teamwork and sharing), and (4) their concern for their own well-being.

THE EVOLVING PATH TO PHYSICIANHOOD

The following pages offer a personal view of the process of medical socialization: the evolving path to physicianhood. The patterns that seem to be part of this process reflect my personal experience in academic medical centers, private general practice settings, house staff programs, and analysis of physician responses to medical education and practice innovations. Social-psychological and medical-sociological writings on medical training have also influenced this perspective.

As an anthropologist, I have been trained to detect examples of ethnocentrism and have internalized a belief structure that values a pluralistic and relativistic world view. As an anthropologist observing the medical co-culture (a contributing segment to other subunits of the American culture), I quickly recognized a species of ethnocentrism. The label "medicocentrism" is a type of ethno-centrism that centrally values medical reality while simultaneously *disvaluing* other realities, such as personalistic, nonorthodox, or spiritual explanations for illness.

Medical ethnocentrism generates a value hierarchy that encompasses both social and technological attributes. For example, the evolving resident values clinical experience (firsthand experience with individual patients and therapies) over generalized, scientific evidence. The resident values the physician's progress note (as the "truth") on a particular patient over that by a nurse or other health professional. The physician values interesting patients/problems (i.e., those that involve diagnostic feats of awe) over common or routine illness experiences or symptoms. The physician values peer recognition over patient recognition (reinforcing physician-derived observations as most valid).

The overriding ideology that becomes internalized as one endures medical education is reductionistic and *scientistic* (partaking of the form of science but not scientific in the sense of valid). The human experience of illness is transformed into the segmented, manageable, episodic character of medical classification, which is a medico-centric reduction of raw data.

Illness is transformed into disease, and disease reflects a disorgan-ized primarily biological mechanism. Correction of this disarray and dysfunction can be accomplished by technological and mechanistic means, or it is simply not valued as part of *appropriate* medical intervention (such as psychiatric or pastoral ministrations). Tech-nology insulates and alienates the patient from the physician as do symbols like white coats — metaphorical extensions of medical machinery. Technology has engineering priests — physicians who become creatures of the superspecialized health shrine — the hospital. Superspecialized technology manipulated by an army of medical personnel may not lead to the best medical care. As one medical educator has summarized this deception of excellence: "Medical practice is needlessly complicated, redundant, ineffective, and, per procedure conducted, inefficient" (Holman quoted in Lander, 1978, p. 86).

How does this ideology become ingrained and perpetuated? What toll does it take on patients and on physicians? What are the mech-anisms that reinforce the medicocentric world view in its dominance, and why is this dominance so obvious at this time in history? These questions are, I believe, crucial, and the responses may help us chart a course that decreases the "thingness" of medical treatment. Other words characterize the same process: dehumanization, mechanization, technologizing, and commodification. It is my thesis that the medicalization process, begun before medical school admission — probably early as nurturance and caring become associated with leadership and physician role models — reinforced in the premed status game (Shulman, 1977), rewarded in medical school activities, and exemplified in the physician role, consolidates during residency. This process produces superb technicians but not flexible providers who can tolerate clinical failure, uncertainty, and ambiguity while maintaining a sense of human value.

MEDICAL STUDENTS

The process of medical education can be a highly discomforting experience. In the first year medical students are confronted with a need to establish a new identity, a need to test themselves in coping with intensive exposure to medical science information, a confrontation with social isolation, and the conflict between mythical expectations and realities. This combination of discrepancies and personal change leads to much perceived stress. I have described medical school as "four years of anxiety waiting for a pill."

Studies published on medical student counseling reveal that most students seek counseling (approximately 60+ percent) at one time or another during their training. When questioned, most medical students feel that 95 percent of their peers would benefit from ongoing counseling. These studies conclude that there is a much greater need for support and/or counseling than is being met in most medical schools. The medical student, even when motivated to seek help or aware of a resource, fears lack of confidentiality, has poor financial resources to pay for aid, and if it is sought perceives counseling as an admission of failure.

Initial medical school years stress "basic" science and a massive cognitive effort. Objectivity and detachment, embedded in biomedical knowledge dominate student culture models. Whether by design or by evolution, affect and empathy are relegated to future periods. Initial medicocentric values thus mirror scientific demeanor. As

Moser (1969) has written, "Our finest academic institutions tend to produce physicians who are so completely preoccupied with the complex liturgy of molecular biology, biochemistry and pathophysiology that they tend to look upon the patient as a curious vessel for the containment of interesting pathology" (p. 809).

On the other hand, the doctor's role must be narrowed and in focus. A perspective too empathic, stimulus receptive, and global will depress the ability to act. Clinical decision making, and the clinical mentality, stress action for its own sake — a curious exaggeration. The medical field that is most closely related to health outcomes, epidemiology, is demeaned as a biostatistical exercise. The prevailing clinical value system supports the argument that population-based knowledge is often inappropriate for individual cases. Epidemiology has few supporters and little positive reinforcement in clinical rotations. Because of this value gap (i.e., the disallowance of epidemiologic thinking), science and medicine begin to be opposites rather than complements.

Beginning medical students who wish to get good grades project memory feats, look "scientific," and try to be calm. They fear the opposite, especially being discovered by patients as being a medical student, contributing to untoward medical harm, making errors, and having a personal health problem. They slowly internalize perfectionistic characteristics, such as perceived personal immunity to disease and a morbid fear of hypochondriasis.

Medical students suffer from sexual and social loneliness. They have few outlets for leisure activities as do their nonmedical age-mates and receive little unqualified friendship. Their faculty tend not to befriend them, and the competitive, independent physician role is used as a defense toward the disillusionment of early physicianhood.

Because clinical integration is an impossible task for basic science teachers and clinicians often fear to coteach with nonmedical researchers, medical students are reinforced in a segmented world view. Clinicians rationalize their discomfortable distance from the "basic science" lecture hall by criticizing the students' poor cognitive base. Students must cope with an apparently unlimited amount of material to learn — with diverse messages from the faculty about what is important and constantly changing and idiosyncratic criteria of what is relevant to later clinical responsibility. Students commonly retreat to particularized study habits that prepare them for exam competency and predispose them to future specialization.

Pathology and disease pathophysiology are the transition courses for the aspiring doctor. The context of disease, either relevant to its population base or to its patient perspective, is assumed to be taught in the clinical years. Unfortunately that assumption is a myth that remains unfulfilled. Students behave and survive by crisis response: a valuable preparation for further segmented medicalization. Their actions are conditioned by immediate objectives: exams.

Medical students attempt to acquire what Fox has called "detached concern," while simultaneously losing much youthful idealism and gaining medical cynicism. Preparation for these medically valued traits occurs in anatomy courses, where cadavers are often nameless and historyless, and in lectures where most topics are intellectualized even if the students' feelings cry out for expression. One surgeon presented a case of penis amputation to a class and then proceeded to display the removed penis with the patient present. Further cynicism and objectification is modeled by case, not patient, presentations. Clinicians model medical discussions as intellectual, scientific pursuits. This pose adaptively shields both the student and the clinician from sickness and suffering. Sickness is, to anthropologists, a social, affective, and moral category, and physicians recognize this by banishing its discussion and concentrating on biomedical disease. Disassociation from sickness is modeled by telescoped phrases that identify the gallbladder in 4 North, the gram-negative meningitis in 6 South, or the code blue (cardiac arrest) in R Wing.

Medical school socialization prepares the student physician for a specialized, technical, and, in the future, high-status world. Student doctors are ideally trained for diagnostic uncertainty, detached concern, limited idealism ("cynicism"), competitiveness, physiochemical primacy and reductionism, and final responsibility.

This training is often brutal and uncoordinated. Training for uncertainty and for the management of finite resources (i.e., the limited time and energy available to the student) is ritualized by negative feedback — scathing criticism — when errors are made or actions are not taken. The student's subjective response to this training is minimized and often denied by intellectualistic arguments.

Coombs (1978) forcefully defends the need for time and faculty commitment to the subjective dimension of all these training experiences. The psychosocial interior of the medical socialization process has been poorly addressed in modern medical training. Coombs notes:

My own interviews and personal observations have clearly revealed the students' unmet need to air, to reflect upon, to emotionally explore, and sort out personal feelings as related to specified developmental tasks. This unfilled need adversely affects students' adjustment in the medical school environment and, no doubt, also lowers the potential quality of patient care. (p. 267)

Medical students emerge from the medical school experience data rich and diagnostically astute. They are, however, unevenly prepared for the consolidating role that graduate medical training demands of them. They have been poorly exposed to medical practice role models, having been oriented primarily by academic and tertiary settings. They have cautiously "tasted" but not "swallowed" responsibility and so are unprepared for the emotional impact it will have on their egos when they are residents. They have been sheltered from the entrepreneurial difficulty of administering a medical role or the personal or financial rewards available from a continuous practice relationship. They have had their ordering and decision-making behavior validated and protected by residents. In their lack of ease they have been minimally comforted by slightly senior physicians — residents, who have not been trained in counseling peers.

RESIDENTS

The most powerful decision maker in the United States is the graduated physician, the individual who has completed at least an internship and/or residency training. The physician's methods of clinical decision making, of communicating with colleagues, and of interacting with patients are largely set during and by the end of residency training.

During the same period, a pattern of denying (a cost of medicalization) the priorities of self, family, and the patient's experience of illness is also firmly entrenched. The full commitment to medicine required by the resident's attendings molds, often for life, the future physician's choice of practice style, approach to medical (and general) problem solving, and unhealthy disregard for personal well-being.

Medical socialization studies concentrate on medical school and foster the impressions that the medical school graduate is a *complete* physician. It is my thesis that professional psychosocial development is accomplished not only in medical school but perhaps even more powerfully in residency and practice settings.

Mumford's (1970) analysis of the internship year compared the differing social contexts for the intern in a university hospital with those in a community hospital setting, with the former socializing the intern for research (and perhaps for a hierarchical role) and specialization and the latter socializing the intern for community practice. The resultant ideologies establish the basis for town-gown controversy, reinforcing a lack of colleagiality.

Miller (1970) focused on the socialization of interns at Harvard and their preparation for an "elite" position in a research or academic career. Miller's study analyzed how interns negotiated the competing demands of the attending faculty, patient care, and the prestigious but future positions available to them because of the Harvard credential. Interns in Miller's book learned more than technical competence. They were socialized to specialty practice and an academic ideology. As the residents negotiated their daily service obligations to their patients, they were manipulated by the promise of future status careers.

Mumford (1970) showed how the norms of the internship settings guided the physician toward particular career options. For example, in the university program, norms associated with the management of clinical uncertainty, "relay learning" (the free exchange of medical information), and "graduated specialization" (specialization will advance medicine) are given high priority. The ingroup within a specialty training track produces its own cohesiveness, protecting its members who get carried away by the "tangents" of generalists. Residents share success and failure. Within the peer confines they are scrutinized mercilessly. Resident scrutiny is powerfully different from scrutiny of medical students in that patient responsibility rests with the residents. For example, one of the most difficult tasks of the chief resident who reviews overnight patient management by the interns is whether to "cover" for a tired intern or not. When an intern has been up all night with six or seven "sick" (medically complex) patients and has forgotten to review a final lab report the chief resident will sometimes interrupt the intern's presentation and retrack it to another area. When an intern has committed a more serious error and the chief resident finds out before the attending physician does, a more difficult situation ensues. Given the call schedules, sleep deprivation, and emotional exhaustion of many residents it is easy to see how peers can both create allegiance and stifle communication with nonspecialty members.

In the community setting, these same norms are given different priorities, preparing the intern for greater interaction with nonspecialist individuals, including both physicians and nonphysicians. Community hospital interns, being in smaller programs, are often by themselves when they see patients and are pushed toward greater reliance on both patient and nonspecialist resources. On the other hand, university interns are part of a "proud company" that pressures them to conform to specialty thinking and insulates them from needing local community (medical and nonmedical) ties.

Bucher's studies on residents in psychiatry and medicine (1965, 1969, 1973) also emphasize the homogenizing influence of the residency setting. She concluded that residents are under pressure to share core behavior, common vocabularies, and modal actions if they are to function effectively in their multipart roles; service, education, and/or research.

The residency experience molds a specialty-specific world view (Bucher, 1973). Its structure is a powerful vehicle for personal and professional identity. The milieu inculcates the attitude that one has not become a physician until one has become accredited in a specialty.

Many studies on residency are critical of it as an institution. They focus on long hours worked by interns (Filanders and Heiman, 1971), the impact of sleep deprivation on detrimental clinical judgments (Friedman, Bigger, and Kornfield, 1971), and the inefficient use of the intern's time (assumedly abused by attendings) (Payson, Gaensler, and Stargardter, 1966; Miller, 1970). Miller (1970) and Mumford (1970) implied that the time required of interns to meet the service and research functions of the teaching hospital often prevents their attainment of educational goals. Thus, competing value priorities enhance the experience of guilt felt by the resident.

The psychological state(s) of interns and residents have been studied, and many anecdotes indicate that they are prone to psychological dysfunction. Valko and Clayton (1975) found that 30 percent of 53 residents in medicine, pediatrics, and surgery had had depression in the internship; the average duration of the depressions was five months (with five lasting almost the entire year). Seven residents had suicidal components, and six with *no* previous marital difficulty had marital problems. The medical, social, and childhood histories of the depressed and nondepressed groups were not significantly different. The majority of the interns were working more than 100 hours per week when their depressions began. None had a significant stressful life event occurring 0 to 30 days prior to the onset of depression. The author speculates that physicians in general have a high rate of depressive illness. Anecdotal evidence on depression is enhanced by the well-known high incidence of emotional illnesses, alcoholism, drug abuse, and suicide among American physicians (Pfifferling, 1980; AMA Department of Mental Health, 1977).

A residency experience that maintains attitudes of dread, dependency, and personal deprivation takes its toll on the health of the healers and, by inference, on their patients. The overriding emotions that are constantly present during medical school are fear, anxiety, insecurity, and frustration. These feelings of dread are somewhat mastered by medical school graduation, only to revivify during internship. Mastery of these feelings is incomplete and coped with by general defensiveness and aggressive individuality.

Medical students and house staff commonly evolve in an environment (the academic setting) that reinforces their dependency status. They are dependent on patients for the few positive strokes they receive, on teachers for essential information on how to be perceived as "mature," on external organizations for obtaining credentials and for licensure, on peers for personal, positive support, and on many other health professionals for learning essential routines in patient care. Constant modeling of dependency on others often produces a role model that cannot foster participative sharing with others.

They are debilitated by social and sleep deprivation; by test and case presentation anxiety; by error and fears, and by feeling in a seemingly eternal student status.

The dread, dependency, and debilitation associated with becoming a physician in most American medical schools poorly prepares the physician for flexibility, an educational and counseling role, and a lifetime confrontation with uncertain decision making.

MECHANISMS OF PERSONAL MEDICALIZATION

How are residents medicalized? They are rewarded by peers, teachers, other health professionals, and patients with accumulating status when they model medicocentric traits.

Residents are evaluated by faculty in relationship to the thoroughness of their historical data gathering in a specialty area, their efficient physical examination, their analytical astuteness in relationship to purported pathophysiology and biochemistry and sometimes their problem-solving ability in arriving at a diagnosis. But they are not taught how to elicit or use the relevant cultural, social, and experiential factors that are part of every illness episode of every patient.

Residents watch their faculty concentrate on patient examples of specific, usually singular, disease categories. They are expected to be current in recent literature on the disease process being discussed. Concomitant patient problems are sloughed over in medical roundsmanship. A glance at any problem-oriented chart will witness that patients rarely have only one problem without synergistic reactions from others; yet, textbooks are written as if only single problems existed and as if this were the way to design therapeutic interventions. Presentations of patient problems rarely, if ever, include socioeconomically relevant data by experts in those areas, and those insights are depreciated if discussed. Patient responses to being the object of rounds are never solicited; thus further insight to personal context is lost.

Residents are medicalized by being symbolically robed in clothing different from attending faculty, student, and patient. They cannot escape from being subdominant to faculty, who completely control their personal discretionary time, yet dominant over patients who are institutionally dressed/ or undressed as the case may be. They are status segregated to eat in the doctors' cafeteria and sleep in the residents' quarters, and it is difficult to socialize apart from their call schedule except with people who are part of the system.

They are medically rewarded for "aggressive" action but not for painstakingly building up the patient's defenses or immunity for the prevention of future disease episodes. Aggressive education tends to generalize into their life-style, reducing further their ability to tolerate other styles of intervention.

Audits of "quality of care" are premised on specific tasks (processes) with immediate results, not on outcomes that are relevant to the overall quality of health that the patient could have. Outcome measurements uniformly are biased because of the unmeasured factors that are "out of the doctor's control." Thus, current quality assurance schemes must "of necessity" reinforce immediacy and action, rather than some potential optimal mix of inaction ("tincture of time") and action.

Residents are further medicalized — in this case, reinforced for being specialty oriented or dependent — by having no sanctioned available time to regularly interact in problem-solving sessions with residents in other fields. For example, the process of learning the benefits and weaknesses of pathologic procedures are privy to pathology residents but only superficially known to those who request them.

Residents are reinforced in their habit of assuming that only physicians' observations are essential by being informally instructed that "when there is little time to read medical record entries read the doctor's notes only." So often, key contextual, patient care data are unavailable. Segmented and poorly coordinated care is fostered by hospital policies that allow separate medical record systems such as nursing notes to coexist with the hospital medical record.

Most case-centered conferences are conducted by a specialty and commonly not with interdisciplinary membership. Rounding, often taking up to half of a resident's day, includes mostly other residents in the same specialty. Less frequently seen in the rounding cycle are attendings of other specialties, and still less frequently are there mixed rounds incorporating other health professionals and specialty trainees. The resident is thus exposed to a homogenizing world view.

THE BENEFITS OF MEDICALIZED TRAINING

Generally speaking, physicians who are rewarded for biologistic reductionism (the core ideology) are superb technicians when a specific diagnosis is made for a specific organ system. When specific treatment modalities are known to be effective they are usually appropriately ordered. Patients who fit into a known organ pathology are superbly cared for by specialized physicians in the United States. Patients with exotic, physical pathologies are "interesting" cases and receive spectacular attention. Diseases that are identifiable, curable, and of short duration receive exemplary care. Diseases that are unknown and appear biologically researchable are most valued as teaching opportunities; they also perpetuate the dominance of the medicocentric model.

Modern American physicians feel that they work best in a technological physician-submissive and specialty-access world. Technology symbolically enhances the purported objectivity that is a hallmark of the "scientific" physician. This precipitates distances between doctor and patient. But needless dependency on "scientific" data denies the application of science to understanding the value of human empathy. Curable and controllable, identified pathology enhances the leadership (the "executive") needs of the scientific physician. Healer and/or nurturant tendencies are suppressed in medical settings that place a priority on physician time and deny the importance of patient time. The physician's often defensive need for omnipotence — enhanced in a medicalized society — is supported in a high status, hierarchical medical center. The humbling effects bestowed by an awareness of medical uncertainty and biological ambiguity are relegated to low status. The medicalized physician loses sight of the healer role, the apostolic function that motivated the decision to become a physician.

Throughout the ebb and flow of these developmental components of physicianhood — objectivity/empathy; caring/curing; healing/disquietude — medicalization conflicts with humanization. It is up to those who recognize the ineffective elements of medical socialization to identify and suggest rehumanization strategies. This chapter has attempted to identify such elements.

CONCLUSION

Professional school should be a supportive, cooperative, joyful place. It should be intellectually nourishing, healthful, and paced at an optimal educational level. Faculty and students should be partners in discovery and decision making. The cruel irony is that training for health professionals is not healthful and that the social and psychological health of its trainees is irrelevant to the school's priorities.

Professional schools should be laced with ecstatic learning experiences, but they are generally not. They are ritual laden, needlessly dependency producing, and often obscurely irrelevant. A majority of clinical experiences available in a teaching hospital are concerned with disease entities that are comparatively rare in community settings. In addition, medical faculty are rewarded for scientific contributions and not for preparing their students for general medical treatment.

Medical school and residency education can be simply described as a set of failed expectations. The trainees expected colleagiality, cooperativeness, and efficient and relevant educational experiences. They found, instead, pressures to be manipulative, competitive, and defensive. They found rituals of roundsmanship, spiced by cruelty ("because I went through it") and much judgmental behavior. They found an unexpected resistance to truth-seeking behavior. They found overburden as a rule and not an environment that stressed problem solving for dealing with an ever-changing clinical uncertainty. They found a value system that extolled the built environment as the most precious resource and not the youthful enthusiasm of the student/resident physician. On all fronts they suffered a crisis of failed expectations.

In a subtle manner young physicians learn to see people almost only through their pathologies and completely miss the resiliency of individuals as they cope with the unexpectedness of the illness. They become medically ethnocentric, wearing what I have called a medicocentric blinder of which they are not aware. They fail to realize that this comparatively closed world view blinds them to the strengths, assets, and recovery images that surround them. They systematically discount hope-enhancing images and skills and fail to realize that the costs of this world view will ultimately reflect not only on their professional group (via anger at the medical system) but also on their personal life-style. A medicocentric vision needlessly reinforces a morbid, overly objectified, mechanistic model of problem solving. They, in turn, cope with personal crises by mechanistic responses, too often reflected in their rates of chemical coping.

Our current mode of medical training brutalizes and dehumanizes a precious human resource: the spirit of the medical trainee. There is no doubt in my mind that most physicians are basically conscientious, compassionate, and altruistic. But medical training denies the person of the doctor. Professional time becomes personal time, and personal time is always secondary to medical time. The person of the physician is removed from many encounters as the professional persona dominates the physician role. This all encompassing ego investment may later take its toll when physicians realize that they are not *only* doctors. The cost to many of the most conscientious and compassionate physicians is reflected in the rates of marital disharmony, suicide, depression and chemical dependency for the medical profession (Pfifferling, 1980). It is a sad paradox that reinforcement of MDeification behavior insulates the physician from a caring and compassionate world. American society confers on its heros elite status and privilege but also denies them their humanity and vulnerability and the chance to receive the revitalizing support they so desperately need.

The medicocentric vision can be reduced if students and residents are exposed to problem-solving techniques that stretch them out of a complacent, reductionistic model. Rounds can be conducted with emphasis on self-care, noninvasive strategies for intervention, and mobilization of patient support networks. Medical students can be examined with reference to alternative problem-solving modalities applied to real patient problems. Young physicians can also be exposed to coping techniques that allow them to go beyond survival in their personal encounter with sustained stress. Virshup, in *Coping in Medical School* (1981), offers an effective self-care plan that models many of these coping insights. If the techniques in this book are available to young physicians, and if they allow faculty and other health professionals to function in a more colleagial environment, we may see the destruction of the medicocentric paradigm.

REFERENCES

American Medical Association, Department of Mental Health. 1977. *Helping the Impaired Physician*. Chicago: American Medical Association.

Becker, M. et al. 1961. *Boys in White: Student Culture in Medical School*. Chicago: University of Chicago Press.

Bucher, P. 1965. The Psychiatric Residency and Professional Socialization. *J. Health Hum. Behavior* 6:197-206.

Bucher, R. et al. 1969. Differential Prior Socialization. *Soc. Forces* 48:213-23.

Bucher, R., and Stelling, J. 1973. Vocabularies of Realism in Professional Socialization. *Soc. Sci. Med.* 7:661-75.

Coombs, R. H. 1978. *Mastering Medicine*. Glencoe, Ill.: Free Press.

Filanders, W., and Heiman, M. 1971. Time Study Comparison of Three Intern Programs. *J. Med. Educ.* 46:142.

Fox, R. 1977. The Medicalization and Demedicalization of American Society. In *Doing Better and Feeling Worse*, ed. J. Knowles. New York: Norton.

Friedman, R. C.; Bigger, J. J.; and Kornfield, S. 1971. The Intern and Sleep Loss. *N. Engl. J. Med.* 285:201-203.

Illich, I. 1976. *Medical Nemesis: The Expropriation of Health*. New York: Pantheon.

Lander, L. 1978. *Defective Medicine*. New York: Farrar, Strauss and Giroux.

Miller, S. J. 1970. *Prescription for Leadership*. Chicago: Aldine.

Mumford, E. 1970. *From Students to Physicians*. Cambridge, Mass.: Harvard University Press.

Payson, H. E.; Gaensler, E. C.; and Stargardter, L. 1966. Time Study of Internship on the University Service. *N. Engl. J. Med.* 264:439-43.

Pfifferling, J. M. 1980. *The Impaired Physician: An Overview*. Chapel Hill, N.C.: Health Sciences Consortium.

Shulman, N. 1977. *Finally I'm a Doctor*. New York: Scribners.

Valko, R. J., and Clayton, P. J. 1975. Depression in Internship. *Dis. Nerv. System* 36:26-29.

Virshup, R. 1981. *Coping in Medical School*. Chapel Hill, N.C.: Health Sciences Consortium.

14

THE MEDICALIZATION OF A PERSON:
A Student Becomes a Physician

Randolph B. Schiffer

Physicians know a number of things, but that alone is not what makes them physicians; otherwise, graduate students would be physicians and standardized board examinations in medicine would measure clinical competence. Rather, an aggregate of certain experiences accounts for the transformation from graduate student to clinician. The ancients knew that physicians need to possess more than mere cognitive knowledge. The ideal medical student was described in the *Samhita*, the Hindu book of medicine, as being "born of a good family, possessed of the desire to learn," and having "strength, energy of action, contentment, character, self-control, a good retentive memory, intellect, courage, purity of mind and body, and a simple and clear comprehension (Levit, 1966). The noncognitive transformation that one experiences in becoming a physician parallels the cognitive process, but it is more difficult for an observer to see and understand. In this chapter I describe some general stages in this noncognitive transformation as I experienced them.

There is an aphorism about the medical center that "everything is downhill after the first two years of medical school." At most medical centers in this country, these first two years are preclinical; the students deal with ideas and facts instead of patients. This is the time when the central cognitive tasks are met in the mastering of biochemistry, physiology, pathology, concepts of disease, and other courses. But students do not *feel* like physicians at this stage, nor do they have much of an idea of how physicians feel. They feel routinized by the unrelenting classroom schedule and isolated from their fellows who sit passively alongside them. They are vaguely apprehensive about the clinical experiences ahead. Will I know enough to be a clinician? Will I be skillful enough? Will I make a mistake? These are apprehensions of preclinical students. It is a time of self-doubt and of waiting for the future.

Graduate school is over when the clinical years of medical school begin, but it takes a variable period of time before this transition is fully felt. This new clinical world of ailing people and their array of caretakers is confusing and unclear. The first clearly new feeling that third-year medical students might experience is that they are no longer alone; they are members of a patient care team in a way that is different from the being-with of graduate students.

> I walked into the hospital five or ten minutes late one morning, early in my third year. Rounds on the internal medicine floor began at 8:00, but I thought I would just join in late. By the time I was through the lobby I had heard my name paged three times and was feeling apprehensive. When I reached my patient care team on clinical rounds, the senior resident was mightily displeased with me. "Rounds start at 8:00 A.M. *Doctor* Schiffer," he said. The "Doctor" was provocative at this point. I would never be late again. I was learning how it felt to be a member of a patient care team. I wasn't sure that this was as much fun as I had expected it to be.

The experience of working as a member of the patient care team and being responsible to that team has many aspects. First, one learns that unreliability and tardiness are more serious than previously. Now, in clinical medicine, one must be where one says one will be and be more or less on time. This is without regard for one's personal preferences about schedules. Soon the clinical medical student learns that this is also without regard for one's feelings. First among all feelings is fatigue.

> My first night "on call" as a medical student on surgery, we operated for 12 hours on a man whose aorta had begun to leak at the site of an aneurysm. This was after a full preceding day's work, including rounds, operations, and admission workups. During the operation I mostly held retractors. When it was over, I felt stiff and dizzy. The sun was just rising as we left the operating room. It was 6:00 A.M. The resident

turned to me and said, "Good thing we're done in time. We have 20 minutes to rest before rounds begin, or you may want to use the time to eat breakfast *and* rest. I wanted to take the day off. But since rounds were in 20 minutes, I went. I was learning that in clinical medicine the patient care jobs take precedence over fatigue.

At first, in medical school, this is exhilarating and exciting. One feels a certain eagerness to "measure up," to meet the standard set by the senior physicians. What a change from the graduate school years just behind!

There is another aphorism about the medical center that cartoons the practical nature of the clinical experience. It is said that a physician need only keep in mind the Three Principles of Clinical Medicine to take care of any patient:

1. If what you're doing is working, keep doing it.
2. If what you're doing is not working, stop doing it.
3. If you don't know what to do, don't do anything.

The joke here concerns the limits of intellection in clinical medicine. Knowing a lot is helpful, but knowing how to act is what keeps a physician out of trouble.

Toward the end of the clinical phase of medical school, in preparation for graduation, medical students begin to experience responsibility for patient care. From the start, this experience is complex.

When I was a senior extern, an "acting intern," an elderly man with heart failure and dementia was admitted. Our service was busy. The senior resident counseled me at the start: "Look Randy, the service is busy. This guy is all yours. You can do whatever you want with him. You can give him IV Lasix; you can get an echocardiogram — whatever you want. But have him off the service by Friday.

The responsibility is *for* the patient's care, but whom is it *to*? Is it to the patient care team and the hospital? to the patient? to the physician? By the end of medical school a student might say that clinical responsibility is for and to the patient but is also beginning to sense that it is not so simple. One works also to maintain one's standing with the care team, the chief resident, the attending physician, the hospital, and the profession.

Graduation from medical school does not make people physicians. One can sign "M.D." after one's name, but there are a host of things one cannot do: prescribe drugs, be a licensed physician, take care of patients. For this, one needs to complete an internship. Before the internship, one does not *feel* like a physician.

> The first day of my internship I walked into the reception area of the pediatric department. I told the secretary that I was one of the new doctors, and asked where I should report. She laughed, and I had to show her my ID card to convince her that I really was one of the new doctors. I laughed, too. I wasn't sure that I was one of the new doctors.

The internship is not a cognitive experience. A smart fourth-year medical student might know as many medical facts as an intern, but interns know how to act like doctors. Interns reexperience the colleagueship of clinical medicine from a position of increased responsibility, and in this they experience the power of the profession to compel certain behaviors.

> Midway through my internship year I was on call for internal medicine. It wasn't until 3:00 A.M. that I made it to the sleeping room and lay down. At 3:20 the phone rang; cardiac arrest on Four West. I sat on the edge of my bed in a stupor. I realized that all I cared about at this point was going back to sleep and that I wasn't really much interested in whether the cardiac patient lived or died. But if I didn't go, what would the medical students think? What would the chief resident think? By this point I was on my way, hoping secretly that the patient would be mercifully and irreparably dead.

The fatigue of internship year is no longer exhilarating. The intern is no longer eager for it but now lives with it as a constant companion. It can be deadening and dulling of interests that had previously been important. Hence, the aphorism that interns only talk with their spouses about two things: what came in the mail and what's for dinner. The fatigue can be an invitation to chronic anger and cynicism.

> I walked into the residents' room one night on call, as "A" intern, and found the "B" intern obviously shaken and upset. "I just slapped a patient, Randy," he said. "He was another one of these old guys who won't answer your questions straight, and I just couldn't stand it when

he kept wandering into stories about his past. I have two more workups
to do tonight, and I just blew up at him for slowing me down."

The volume of the work, the hours, the exhaustion — this experience makes it possible for interns to learn detachment in clinical
work. In the beginning, the suffering of the seriously ill and their
families is fearful and anxious for student physicians. It can even
mesmerize and paralyze clinicians if they are unable to separate
themselves from it. Interns learn that it is just not physically possible to get caught up in the anguish of so many patients.

On the last night of my year a woman was dying a respiratory death,
with her family in attendance. She was on IV bronchodilators, steroids,
and adrenergic drugs, plus antibiotics and inhalation therapy. Still her
gasping continued, and it became obvious that she was worsening. I
checked the IV lines and the mist mask and made some minor adjustments in the drug dosages. I sat for 15 minutes with the family. One
daughter wept the whole time. The husband asked several questions,
and I told him as much as we knew. I left to go to bed but was stopped
by the third-year medical student who said in disbelief: "How can you
go to bed? How can you sleep while this patient is dying? Don't you
care?" I cared. But I was also tired. And I also felt confident of myself
now; confident that everything possible was being done for this woman.
I knew I would be called when something changed.

As one becomes slowly more comfortable and familiar with the
anguish of the patients, one finds a gradual decrement of one's own
anxiety. The clinical situations and decisions multiply themselves
again and again, and then they feel familiar. In place of the earlier
doubts and anxieties, intern clinicians may be aware of a sense of
mastery over their responses. This is preliminary, of course, and far
from the more complete mastery of senior residents or attending
physicians. But it is a reassuring feeling of knowing what to do and
how to do it in most difficult situations, at least during the time
while one waits for definitive help. This sense does not emerge
from learning facts and research, although much of this learning is
occurring as well. It emerges from experiencing sick people over a
prolonged period of time — the way they look and the way they feel
and sound. After enough of this one knows in a practical way what
needs to be done. Sometimes this new sense of being a physician
is first experienced through the responses of those around. It may be
in a look or in a question.

One night they brought a 10-month-old girl to the emergency room after her parents found her apparently dead in her crib. I was paged "Stat" to the emergency room and ran all the way. There was the usual confusion — nurses wheeling carts about, the distraught parents, a surgical intern starting cardiopulmonary resuscitation on the still, pale infant. As the only pediatric house officer in the hospital, I was in charge, although I was not directly aware of this. For me, there was only the situation, the faces turned toward me waiting, and the things to be done: parents out (nothing they can help with now), ambu bag, EKG on, IV in, NaH_2CO_3 injection, heart activity?, defibrillate 30 watt seconds shock, recheck EKG, and on and on. Afterward it occurred to me that people in this hospital no longer asked to see my ID card, and I no longer felt like I needed to show it.

There is more to the noncognitive development of the physician than I have been able to tell here. But these are some of the experiences that go into it: the fatigue, responsibility, detachment, and the beginnings of mastery.

REFERENCE

Levit, L. P. 1966. The Personality of the Medical Student. *Chicago Med. School Q.* 25:201-14.

PART IV

Too Much or Too Little Medicalization

The concern of Illich that medicine has expanded its domain and expropriated activities and responsibilities better left to others is echoed in Chapter 15 by Brown, who finds in the present behavior of Western physicians a situation reminiscent of the Medical Police proposed in the late eighteenth century in Germany by J. P. Frank. These proposals, Brown argues, were aimed at professional aggrandizement for gains in power, influence, personal gratification, and perhaps income. He views the institutionalization of tuberculous patients in the same light. By contrast, Ciaglia, in Chapter 16, sees too little medicalization in the failure of physicians to adequately care for the chronically ill, creating a vacuum into which a multitude of voluntary health agencies have moved. What is needed is an increased involvement of medicine in the comprehensive, long-term care needs of chronically ill patients. There is almost a suggestion of the need to move toward a more holistic form of health care, not limited to the strictly biomedical components of health care.

Some observers detect a form of Western medicalization in developing countries. In Chapter 17, Bijleveld and Varkevisser note examples of imprudent promotion of Western technology in East Africa, but they believe the overwhelming problem is a lack of sufficient technology in the form of better regimens for dealing with widespread infectious disease. They find too *little* medicalization in the attack on leprosy and tuberculosis.

There is, then, a sharp division of interpretation on whether medical care is overly expansionist with an emphasis on a need for a more comprehensive, caring medical system.

15

J. P. FRANK'S "MEDICAL POLICE" AND ITS SIGNIFICANCE FOR MEDICALIZATION IN AMERICA

Theodore M. Brown

"Medicalization by taxonomic expansion" is a process which Janzen, in Chapter 1, views as separable from the "increasing control of medicine by state and professional bureaucracies." By distinguishing sharply between belief systems and the instruments of state he has argued provocatively for the positive evaluation of taxonomic extension, thus distancing himself from a number of other scholars who view the widening of "medical" categories in the popular culture as a cause for alarm. The sociologist Irving Zola, for example, points to an important anomaly: medicalizing many problems does not really serve effectively to destigmatize them. Rather, despite hopes to the contrary, the metaphor of illness by itself seems to provide no release from individual responsibility or moral judgment. Indeed, the shift in the handling of such problems is "primarily in those who will undertake the change . . . and where the change will take place. . . . The problem being scrutinized and the person being charged is no less immoral for all the medical rhetoric" (Zola, 1975, p. 87). A pernicious form of victim-blaming in which victims readily blame themselves seems to follow the expansion of medical taxa.

Another very large set of issues lies behind the apparent willing extension of medical categories by the "lay public." For how much that is apparent here is real? How much unseen inspiration and hidden manipulation lie behind the perhaps deceptive facade of appearances? What larger social forces – economic, political, and cultural – may be needed to explain medicalization in a particular stratum of society at a particular point in time? Lasch (1977) has written about a rapidly expanding "religion of health" in nineteenth century Europe and America that followed on the advent of capitalism and the rise of bourgeois society. Nor did this new religion merely "evolve," although many in society *seemed* drawn to it freely and spontaneously. Rather, it was "imposed" on society by the "forces of organized virtue," while doctors in particular advanced the "medical mode of salvation . . . hand in hand with the state" (pp. 169-70). As it was in the nineteenth century so it may be in the twentieth: it is possible that the public is taking most of its cues from the professionals.

My purpose here is to focus on only one feature of what seems to be a very complex process that involves, at the very least, economic forces, political ideology, popular culture, and professional aggrandizement. The feature on which I will focus is professional aggrandizement, an aggradizement that proceeds from the "top down" along with whatever "bottom up" features of medicalization move upward simultaneously. My basic claim is that in any instance of supposed medicalization it is both instructive and important to look for the possible role of professional aggrandizement without, however, using it to deny the influence of other forces and circumstances.

To advance this claim succinctly but (it is hoped) effectively, I have chosen to present two parallel case examples, one from turn-of-nineteenth century Germany and another from turn-of-twentieth century America. I will also argue that these two examples relate not only by strategic parallelism but by direct descent. Naturally, given our time constraints, I can only present here the bare outlines of much richer case materials.

Let us consider first the medical profession in late eighteenth century Europe. Although it is, of course, an enormously oversimplified generalization, it seems safe to say that the European medical profession at this time was in serious trouble. The suspicion of medicine's therapeutic inefficacy, indeed of its outright harmfulness, had spread rapidly and widely by midcentury. European physicians, long regarded with considerable skepticism, by 1750 faced criticism whose frequency, intensity, and acidity had greatly increased. The French *Encyclopédie*, for example, displayed clearly a strong current of antiprofessional, self-help, and hygienic sentiment

(Coleman, 1974). The appearance of this sentiment paralleled changed attitudes in the literature on "population," an eighteenth century European obsession. Whereas earlier political economists had included calculations of the precise number of physicians necessary for optimal human breeding conditions, those of the latter eighteenth century tended to pass over doctors and to recommend direct interventions in the physical environment instead (Rosen, 1974). In 1762 Rousseau captured and crystallized an increasingly popular mood when he wrote in *Emile*:

> . . . against one life saved by the doctors you must set a hundred slain . . . I do not deny that medicine is useful to some men; I assert that it is fatal to mankind. . . . Hygiene is the only useful part of medicine, and hygiene is rather a virtue than a science. (1972, pp. 21-23)

In these circumstances it was not surprising to find many physicians trying to co-opt the rapidly growing lay hygiene movement. Thus, in 1762 Dr. John Fothergill added still another health manual to the ample supply already available. This one, the reader is told by the subtitle, contains "All that has been recommended by the most eminent Physicians." The fulsome dedication to the "Worshipful College of Physicians" of London praises a medical society deeply concerned about "Rules for the Preservation of Health." In France, the founding of the Royal Society of Medicine in 1778 seems to grow out of the same co-optive political motives. To make themselves useful to the state, this vanguard group of physicians forged an alliance with progressive elements in the French bureaucracy. The new medical society agreed to perform administrative duties in exchange for recognition as the authoritative agency recommending national policy in preventive medicine (Hannaway, 1972).

In Germany, the environment in which J. P. Frank created his *System of a Complete Medical Police* (6 volumes, 1779-1817), circumstances were very different from those either in England or France. Consequently, neither Fothergill's nor the Royal Society of Medicine's co-optive strategies were readily available to physicians. Instead, Frank (our symbol of a larger German movement) had to build his *System* of detailed "womb to tomb" health regulations from elements of eighteenth century "cameralism".

"Cameralism" was the carefully articulated system of German rational statecraft that included among its subdivisions mercantilist regulation of commerce and finance and "police" supervision of domestic and internal security (Rosen, 1974). Construing the police authority widely, cameralists argued that the state could intrude into almost every area of life: prescribing sanitary regulation, supervising public entertainments, mandating proper "eugenic" marriage policies, and recommending dress codes. Long before Frank was born, *Polizey* had been accorded extensive treatment in massive academic tomes on cameralistic science, a subject institutionalized through the creation of special chairs at several German universities. Since matters pertaining to health and medicine were a regular feature of "Polizey" throughout the eighteenth century, it was in no way extraordinary that Joseph von Sonnenfels, the cameralistic authority on whom Frank relied most extensively, devoted considerable attention to medical and public health regulation in his multivolume textbook (Sonnenfels, 1765). When putting together his own *System*, Frank tried to separate and transform the "Gesundheitspolizey" thread already in cameralism.

This separation and transformation, then, was Frank's special German version of the common co-optive strategy of later eighteenth century European physicians. Since German jurists and bureaucrats already had claim to the "health" area, considered crucial for population growth and economic development, they were not willing to form an alliance with physicians, as were the French. Frank therefore had to medicalize cameralistic health policy, that is, literally convert existing *Gesundheitspolizey* into *Medicinischepolizey*. By doing so he knew he would earn "the envy of jurists, who were used for centuries to be exclusively in charge of matters of state" (p. 307). But it was worth suffering personal recrimination if by doing so "the influence of medical science on the well-being of the states would attain a new splendor . . . and that physicians would cease to be regarded as men who are only more or less successful in making others healthy" (p. 4).

Frank's aim, in other words, was to restore physicians to proper regard by widening their role to include the field of prescribed prevention. To establish physicians firmly in that field in Germany required the displacement of jurists and administrators. To accomplish this, Frank had to invoke *medical science* as a new basis for authoritative judgment in health matters.

Ideally, Frank thought, medicine could achieve a new dominance. Humanity, or at least humanity's enlightened rulers, might come to realize that medical science had made considerable progress in recent years. Mortality from several diseases had declined, and "does this not permit us to conclude that the cause of this decrease lies in the progress of medical and surgical science?" (p. 298). Likewise, advances in obstetrics had resulted in significantly lower infant and maternal mortality and the pharmacopoeia had been greatly improved. Even in conditions that medicine could not yet cure, it was able to reduce the duration and hence the expense of illness and it could certainly mitigate pain and suffering. All these accomplishments, Frank believed, justified the extension of medicine into the sphere of the jurists, where the physician's expertise would immeasurably improve the drafting of medical police ordinances. For example:

> If the healthy situation of a place were the only criterion decisive for the settlement of a human society in some region or other, the physician — who would use all his experience of climate and the confluence of unfavorable physical causes of exhausted nations, as well as the principles of a rational knowledge of air, water, and soil — could stipulate many beneficial rules according to which people should act in founding new towns and establishing new colonies. (p. 175)

Or again, and more generally,

> . . . chiefly the physician should be heard because it can be expected only of him that, in addition to accurate knowledge of the human body, he also knows the relationship of the causes which affect it, and only he is able to discover the manifold springs [of human life] which have many sources, and the drying up of which is not always the unalterable fate of mortals. (p. 201)

If Frank were to have his way, the physician would become the unchallenged, expert guide to the health of the state. Justifying this authority by appealing to presumably esoteric medical science (primarily physiology and some anatomy), Frank sought thus to displace blame from the physician's suspect therapy to corrupt society and to assure medical practitioners professional recognition as managers of preventive practice. In every area of their lives and in every corner of society, people should be *forced* to maintain or improve their health. Physicians, Frank showed, were prepared to take the lead in drafting the police regulations.

In the United States in the latter nineteenth century circumstances for the medical profession were strikingly parallel to those that had prevailed in late eighteenth century Europe. Although this, too, is a greatly oversimplified generalization, it seems safe to say that the American medical profession in the late nineteenth century found itself in awful circumstances (Rothstein, 1972). The ranks of the profession were overcrowded and divided into rival sects. A popular hygiene movement and various health cults challenged professional practice of any kind. Incompetent faculties of proprietary schools poured inadequately trained graduates into an already flooded market, while the popular press condemned medical graduates of all kinds, whether of proprietary schools or not. Shryock (1936) has summarized press reaction as follows:

> . . . [the *Elmira Gazette* for May 20, 1879] announced that doctors tried to keep their patients ill. In New York City a citizen died after treatment by a specialist, whereupon *Harper's Weekly* [for February 5, 1859] carried long and agonizing accounts, including drawings illustrating the case. One of the large dailies waxed so indignant that it declared the entire medical guild a "stupendous humbug. (p. 253)

The one sphere of action in which physicians participated with general approval was public health. Public health had emerged as a national concern just before the Civil War, drew major attention during it, and attained institutionalization with the creation of the American Public Health Association a few years after its conclusion (Ravenel, 1921). Public health activities had many motives in those decades: guarding against or at least limiting epidemic disease, producing a healthy work force for rapidly industrializing America, and socializing the immigrant masses (Brown, 1979). Physicians participated in all phases of this activity, but as Rosenkrantz (1974) has written, "while the participation of the professional physician was paramount, there was the clear sense that his contribution lay less in his scientific acumen than in his responsible citizenship" (p. 58). Thus, despite their intimate association with it, physicians could still not claim public health work as a specifically *medical* activity. Authority distributed horizontally at best, with vanguard physicians serving, at the most, on par with lay advocates for public health action.

Horizontal distribution of authority persisted despite the growing respect for "science" and "professionalism" in late nineteenth

century American middle class culture (Bledstein, 1976). The principal reason for this was that the "science" of public health was clearly
accessible to intelligent laymen. It was a mixture of sanitary ideas
and civil engineering, "miasmatic" speculation, and generalized
physiology, already widely diffused in the popular culture through
such books as Beecher's *Letters to the People on Health and Happiness* (1855). Since it was eclectic and decidedly nonesoteric, the
"science" of public health could not be claimed as the exclusive
possession of physician-professionals.

Bacteriology, however, was an entirely different matter. This
science, which grew rapidly in Europe in the 1870s and 1880s, was
a most complex and difficult new field. To command it, one needed
to be expert in sophisticated solid media culture techniques, staining,
and microscopy. Bacteriology also proved strikingly successful in
rapidly identifying the causative organisms responsible for major
epidemic and endemic diseases — cholera and tuberculosis to name
just two. As a science that worked and as a science that was at the
same time unquestionably esoteric, bacteriology exercised a strong
attraction on certain leading members of the American medical
profession. They gravitated toward it and began to apply it as Frank
had earlier applied physiology. With bacteriology in their exclusive
possession, physicians for the first time could exert a true dominance
over the field of public health. With bacteriology they could medicalize public health practice, and, thus medicalized, public health
could assure physicians the status they sought.

The impact of bacteriology on American public health was
indeed dramatic. Already in the 1870s the popular press reflected the
tensions in the public health movement between physicians who
stressed particular diseases and sanitarians who favored general
cleanup campaigns and broad social reforms. *Leslie's Illustrated
Weekly* reacted to a warning about a possible relapsing fever
epidemic by charging that doctors were trying to create a panic
"simply to magnify the imaginary services of a physician" (Duffy,
1974, p. 49). These suspicions proved prescient, for at the turn of
the twentieth century Joseph McCormack, retained in 1900 by the
American Medical Association literally to "organize" the medical
profession, repeatedly chastized the public for its failure to follow
the "enlightened guidance of physicians in areas only they could
understand" (Burrow, 1977, p. 21). Thoroughly committed to the
new bacteriology, McCormack, a former secretary of the Kentucky

State Board of Health, consistently advanced the claims of expert physicians over those of lay sanitarians in his whistle-stop campaign around the country. Only bacteriologically competent physicians could organize proper preventive measures, which were capable of stopping the spread of tuberculosis, typhoid, diphtheria, scarlet fever, and cholera infantum. Finally, in 1915 Charles V. Chapin, health officer of Providence, Rhode Island, and later chief spokesman for public health within the American Medical Association, consolidated the status of bacteriologist-physicians within the public health movement by assigning appropriate numerical values to various "lines of health work" (Chapin, 1934, pp. 37-45). On a scale of 100, medical inspection for communicable diseases was worth 13 and antituberculosis activities 10, whereas garbage removal and clean-up campaigns were each worth 0.

Flexner's *Medical Education in the United States and Canada* (1910), commissioned by the Carnegie Foundation, probably most effectively projected the definitive image of the bacteriologically transformed physician. In several passages Flexner describes the new American physician as an arm of the state, an "organ differentiated by society for its own highest purposes" as a means of promoting health, physical vigor, and social peace (p. 19). "Upon him," he wrote, "society relies to ascertain, and through measures essentially educational to enforce, the conditions that prevent disease and make positively for physical and moral well-being" (p. 26). Society's faith is well placed, for "modern hygiene, largely the outcome of bacteriology, has elevated the physician from a mainly personal to a mainly social status" (p. 67). Or, in slightly different words,

> Thus the laboratory sciences all culminate and come together in the hygienic laboratory; out of which emerges the young physician, equipped with sound views as to the nature, causation, spread, prevention, and cure of disease, and with an exalted conception of his own duty to promote social conditions that conduce to physical well-being. (p. 68)

Parallel to Frank's physician but with adjusted means for altered circumstances, the new American physician was prepared to enjoy the recognition that came with dominance over a field of established public esteem.

Thus far we have dealt only with parallels between "Medical Police" and "Bacteriological Hygiene." It is also possible, however, to suggest direct linkages between these two instances of medical-professional aggrandizement. These linkages connect Frank with Flexner via the continued evolution of "Medical Police" in nineteenth-century Germany.

A quick glimpse of that evolution reveals two major developmental stages, essentially pre- and post-Bismarck. In the earlier stage, "medical police" grew largely as a part of regulative domestic bureaucratic machinery. In a tiered hierarchy ultimately responsible to the Minister of the Interior, salaried "medical police" officers administered medical care, monitored epidemics, collected precise, detailed information on agriculture and the human population, and enforced mandatory vaccination. Furthermore, medical police officers were required to "inspect the shops of apothecaries, and superintend the medical topography of . . . [the] district, the pauper medical relief, and all public hospitals, baths, schools, prisons, etc., with reference to their hygienic condition" (*Westminster Review*, 1846, pp. 72-73). In the later, post-Bismarck developmental stage, "medical police" was transformed into modern bacteriological public health at the service of the imperial state. Mandatory vaccination, compulsory bacteriological diagnosis, and forced confinement of the microbiologically impure, whether in specially constructed barracks or in more beneficent-seeming sanatoria, were the later techniques of police control backed by full military authority. German imperial officials applied medical police powers in this form in both colonial and domestic settings (Palmberg, 1893; Dolman, 1973).

Turn-of-twentieth century American physicians picked up German medical police in this latter form. Earlier American public health figures — John Griscom (1845) and Lemuel Shattuck (1850), for example — had reacted quite positively to the first version of German medical police, and some 50 or so years later Hermann Biggs (1902) and William Henry Welch (1920) responded enthusiastically to the second. Biggs, for example, campaigned vigorously for mandatory tuberculosis registration. Required bacteriological examination of sputum samples would be the principal means of identifying and verifying presence of the disease. Philadelphia physicians were quite right to note that the policy Biggs pushed in New York would, if implemented in their own city, represent an intrusion of a new, "German" style of public health (Rosenkrantz, 1974). For his own part, Welch, Dean at Johns Hopkins and a central figure in American medicine, actively campaigned for the German model. When he came to Albany, New York, in 1908 to help launch a statewide anti-tuberculosis campaign, he told his audience:

> In Germany today some twenty-five thousand patients in the early stages of tuberculosis are treated in sanatoria . . . [but there is also another important institution] the special tuberculosis dispensary. . . . The German conception of this institution is expressed by the designation "information aid station." (1920, vol. 1, pp. 634-35)

The idea of regulating the tuberculous poor by confining them to special institutions and then controlling every aspect of their lives had already surfaced in America. Consider the following remarks in the 1890 issue of the *Journal of the American Medical Association*:

> A phthisical patient should have every act of his life, every breath he draws or mouthful of food he eats, his exercise, his rest, in a word all his habits regulated by a skilled physician. And only in a well conducted institution can he be thus managed. Of the encouraging results that can be accomplished by such sanitaria witness those of Europe, notably those of Goebersdorf and Frankinstein in the inclement climate of Germany. (p. 276)

American physicians' enthusiasm for the transformed "medical police" package in which German bacteriology came wrapped seems readily explicable in terms of the social rationalization and social control functions to which many in turn-of-twentieth century America gravitated. A new rational order in which the bacteriologist-physician served as a principal, perhaps *the* principal, social engineer had obvious appeal to a profession trying to elevate and consolidate its status. Like Frank trying to fit into yet take over cameralism, American bacteriological physicians were eager to demonstrate their social utility while simultaneously striving to come out atop the professional heap.

What, then, were the consequences of this act of professional aggrandizement. For those people who were mostly poor and diagnosed as microbiologically impure, professional aggrandizement meant stigmatization and, possibly, institutional confinement. Whereas previously, poor immigrant consumptives might have suffered amidst family, now they were sought out with the latest instruments of medical science and forced into sanatoria. Aggregate environments were left unreformed while individual victims of disease entities seen only by professionals were put under strict supervision. And with the presumed goal of finding ever more "germs," public health officials imposed strict quarantine at the ports and then entered the schools. Once in the schools, the scope of medical interest and the range of medical supervision rapidly increased. As Burrow (1977) writes in his *Organized Medicine in the Progressive Era*:

> The movement for medical inspection, which had as its original goal the prevention of the spread of contagious diseases, broadened its objectives after the new century began. . . . Cornelius C. Wholey, a Pittsburgh physician, suggested that efforts should be made to detect any . . . mental or physical defects and to investigate the hygienic condition of the school environment. (pp. 93-94)

Here is a specific instance of the expansion of medical taxa by physicians exploiting what Freidson (1970) has called the "halo effect" of bacteriology. Because of the sacred glow surrounding bacteriological success, physicians apparently felt justified in expanding their area of concern to include mental health, and, ultimately, the school environment in general. They had successfully insinuated themselves into a larger sphere, and there they lingered even when direct bacteriological concerns disappeared.

REFERENCES

Beecher, C. 1855. *Letters to the People on Health and Happiness*. New York: Arno Press (Facsimile reprint, 1972).

Biggs, H. 1902. Sanitary Measures for the Prevention of Tuberculosis in New York City and Their Results. *J.A.M.A.* 39:1635-40.

Bledstein, B. 1976. *The Culture of Professionalism*. New York: Norton.

Brown, E. R. 1979. *Rockefeller Medicine Men: Medicine and Capitalism in America*. Berkeley: University of California Press.

Burrow, J. G. 1977. *Organized Medicine in the Progressive Era*. Baltimore: Johns Hopkins University Press.

Chapin, C. V. 1934. *Papers*. New York: The Commonwealth Fund.

Coleman, W. 1974. Health and Hygiene in the *Encyclopédie*: A Medical Doctrine for the Bourgeoisie. *J. History Med.* 29:399-421.

Dolman, C. 1973. Robert Koch. In *Dictionary of Scientific Biography*, vol. 7, ed. C. C. Gillispie, pp. 420-35. New York: Scribners.

Duffy, J. 1974. *A History of Public Health in New York City, 1866-1966*. New York: Russell Sage Foundation.

Flexner, A. 1910. *Medical Education in the United States and Canada: A Report to the Carnegie Foundation*. New York: The Carnegie Foundation.

Fothergill, J. 1762. *Rules for the Preservation of Health: Containing all that has been Recommended by the most Eminent Physicians*. London.

Frank, J. P. 1779-1817. *A System of Complete Medical Police*, 6 vols. Reprinted 1976, ed. E. Lesky, Baltimore: Johns Hopkins University Press.

Freidson, E. 1970. *Profession of Medicine*. New York: Dodd, Mead.

Griscom, J. 1845. *The Sanitary Condition of the Labouring Class of New York*. New York: Arno Press (facsimile reprint, 1970).

Hannaway, C. 1972. The Société Royale de Médecine and Epidemics in the Ancien Regime. *Bull. History Med.* 46:257-73.

Lasch, C. 1977. *Haven in a Heartless World*. New York: Basic Books.

Medical Police of the United Kingdom. 1846. *Westminister Review* 45:56-88.

Palmberg, A. 1893. *A Treatise on Public Health and its Applications in Different European Countries*, trans. A. Newsholme. Hamburg: Sonnen Scheen.

Ravenel, M. 1921. *A Half Century of Public Health*. New York: APMA.

Rosen, G. 1974. *From Medical Police to Social Medicine*. New York: Science History Publications.

Rosenkrantz, B. G. 1974. Cart before Horse: Theory, Practice and Professional Image in American Public Health, 1870-1920. *J. History Med.* 29:55-73.

Rothstein, W. 1972. *American Physicians in the Nineteenth Century*. Baltimore: Johns Hopkins University Press.

Rousseau, J. J. 1762. *Emile*. Reprinted 1972, trans. B. Foxley. London: Dent.

Sanitaria for the Consumptive Poor. 1890. *J.A.M.A.* 14:276-77.

Shattuck, L. 1850. *Report of the Sanitary Commission of Massachusetts*. Boston: Harvard University Press, 1948.

Shryock, R. H. 1936. The *Development of Modern Medicine*. Philadelphia: University of Pennsylvania Press.

Sonnenfels, J. von. 1765. *Grundsätze der Polizey, Handlung und Finanz*. Vienna.

Welch, W. H. 1920. *Papers and Addresses*. 3 vols. Baltimore: Johns Hopkins University Press.

Zola, I. K. 1975. In the Name of Health and Illness: On Some Socio-Political Consequences of Medical Influence. *Soc. Sci. Med.* 9:83-87.

16

MEDICALIZATION:
A Boon to the Care Needs of
People with Chronic Health Problems

Donald J. Ciaglia

From a broader, more positive perspective and definition, medicalization might be considered as the "care" component of the
physician's "cure-care" armamentarium and as such would be
heralded as a medical advance by those people and their families
burdened by what McKeown (1976) describes as the "residual health
problems to be found in technologically advanced countries" and a
host of other chronic health problems. To be sure, an echo of
acclaim would also be heard from the army of American voluntary
health agencies (VHAs) that in the main address gaps and leakages
in the traditional health delivery system and which have, through
default of the medical profession, assumed the care responsibility
for those with chronic, long-term care health needs. A glance at
listings of a community's voluntary health agencies (e.g., Multiple
Sclerosis Association, Cerebral Palsy Association, Retarded Children
Association) readily supports this.

The voluntary health agency industry is big business. It is con-
servatively estimated that there are presently in excess of 36,000
local, state, and national organizations providing essential health
care services for tens of thousands of chronically ill people. Total
budget estimates range from three to ten billion dollars annually.
In addition, the VHAs continue to serve as catalysts in focusing
public attention and financial support for a myriad of health problems. Although it is becoming increasingly more complicated to

differentiate between the voluntary and public health systems, and despite predications of Ford (1976) and others that "the advent of federal financing of health services and community health planning in the past decade has weakened the influence of voluntary health organizations and raised doubts about their future direction," the voluntary health agency industry continues to flourish. The continuing success of VHAs might well be attributed to a number of national political and social influences embedded in an early history of American volunteerism. Schlesinger (1953, p. 3) described this "philanthropic streak" as "another of the distinguishing marks of the American Way," while the National Commission on Community Health Services (1966, p. 6) reported that "Volunteerism has overtones and undertones of business and social status for many people, reflecting a subjective phenomenon difficult for either behavioral scientists and politicians to assess. Such voluntary citizen participation is one of the most dynamic resources available in a democracy. The responsibility of government, however, is simply to preserve and insure an atmosphere in which volunteerism can flourish."

In view of the apparently healthy financial and organizational growth pattern and projected survival status of the VHA industry, one might logically question the merits of realignment of VHAs with what Illich (1976) considers to be a major threat to health — the medical establishment. The answer pragmatically rests in terms of *reality*: *reality* colored by social, political, and economic influences; the *reality* of a belief that the continued limited involvement of the medical profession with the chronic care and personal service needs of the clients of VHAs would truly represent a "nemesis"; the *reality* that a broader perspective and definition of medicalization that "supports a more integrated and reciprocal relationship between a society and its medical system" (de Vries, 1978) would enhance the welfare of people with residual health problems to a greater degree than would the philosophy that "the society which can reduce professional intervention to a minimum will provide the best conditions for health" (Illich, 1976, p. 123).

Contrary to Carlson's (1975, p. 143) declaration "we have the medicine we deserve," clients of VHAs do not deserve the medicine (or lack of) they have been receiving. Once the acute phase of a condition with all its implication of highs (technology, cost, and physician's interest) wanes and chronicity sets in, a robotlike exodus of physician involvement (demedicalization) takes place. Referrals to the next level of care, usually a VHA, are all too often accomplished with a minimum, if any, of physician input. The concept of a continuum of care becomes illusory between the acute and chronic stages of diseases. And once a placement has been made, follow-up by the referring physician becomes a rare phenomenon. If a broader implication of medicalization insures a physician's expanded concern for a patient regardless of the stage of illness or site of care, this would indeed be considered as medical advance in the eyes of the chronically ill. For as Eisenberg (1977, p. 236) states "In a sense, the mere presence of a doctor is the medicine." These clients are not the worried well but rather the confirmed disabled. Nor is the medicalization process "the progressive annexation of not illness into illness" (Sedgwick, 1973, p. 37). Medicalization in this instance equates with good, sound, humanistic medicine with a potential for a positive psychological impact far outweighing the risk of dependency.

Probably no other group possesses more first-hand experience and knowledge of the limitations of the biotechnological capacities of physicians while still recognizing the symbolic power of their actions than do VHAs and their clients. Regardless of their self-limited involvement with VHAs, physicians still serve as the main brokers of health services with signatory privileges. "He is the gatekeeper to the production of medical care" (Fuchs, 1974, p. 57); and this captain of the team role extends currently into the arena of the VHAs. An increased medicalization posture holds promise that the "captain" might well be willing to take a turn at bat in the "care" game. The inculcation of this broadened perspective of medicalization will need to be achieved through innovative changes in medical education, including both curriculum and settings. Utilizing community health agencies as a laboratory early in medical education is an effective means of nurturing the care interests of physicians.

To advocate the expanded role of physicians in the care of the chronically ill solely on the basis of symbolic power would be a travesty. That is the current state of the art. What is needed is a physician's "commitment to care" to health problems and in settings that often lack the incentives of intellectual, emotional, and financial rewards inherent in acute, curative, high-cost, hospital-based medicine. There is a need to bring to the VHAs the physicians' capability to perform a care function — a function that physicians have traditionally filled in other settings — a function that is due to the "decline of religious belief, the breakup of families, the increase in mobility and anonymity in our urban culture, and the complexities of psychosocial problems associated with chronic illness. "It may well be that the demand for 'caring' is greater than ever before" (Fuchs, 1974, p. 65).

No doubt the issue of medicalization will continue to be debated with increasing fervor. Fox (1977) has clearly enunciated the parameters of the battle. In the meantime political, social, and economic forces appear to be leading us into some form of national health insurance with promises of comprehensive health care. Will this comprehensive health care provide for all? Traditionally health plans have paid for "those things doctors do." Will the current limited role (demedicalization) that physicians play in VHA programs preclude the chronically ill from receiving benefits? Or will an expanded physician role (medicalization) at long last focus in on the needs of those with residual health problems? In the final analysis, this reality overshadows the philosophical issues.

REFERENCES

Carlson, R. J. 1975. *The End of Medicine.* New York: Wiley-Interscience.

de Vries, M. 1978. Opening Comments at Conference on Medicalization. Rochester, New York.

Eisenberg, L. 1977. The Search for Care. In *Doing Better and Feeling Worse,* ed. J. Knowles. New York: Norton.

Ford, A. 1976. *Urban Health in America.* Oxford: Oxford University Press.

Fox, R. 1977. The Medicalization and Demedicalization of American Society. In *Doing Better and Feeling Worse,* ed. J. Knowles. New York: Norton.

Fuchs, V. 1974. *Who Shall Live?* New York: Basic Books.

Illich, I. 1976. *Medical Nemesis: The Expropriation of Health.* New York: Pantheon.

McKeown, T. 1976. *The Role of Medicine: Dream, Mirage, or Nemesis?* Princeton, N.J.: Princeton University Press.

National Commission on Community Health Services. 1966. *Health Is a Community Affair.* Cambridge, Mass.: Harvard University Press.

Sedgwick, P. 1973. Illness: Mental and Otherwise. *The Hastings Center Studies.* 1(3):19-40.

Schlesinger, A., Sr. 1953. The True American Way of Life. *St. Louis Post Dispatch.*

17

LEPROSY CONTROL IN EAST AFRICA:
Medicalization in Developing Countries

Iman Bijleveld
Corlien M. Varkevisser

In many developing countries the introduction of "Western" or, as we tend to call them, "modern" medical practices and products is of recent origin. It has not happened in isolation but rather as part of a process of change involving the introduction of many different kinds of technologies. This development may expose residents of these developing countries to the medicalization that Illich (1976) describes in Western societies.

Examples of excessive or inappropriate use of modern medical technology in developing countries already abound. The extension of health services has inevitably attracted people with complaints that without intervention would soon have disappeared. Even in such instances the administration of antibiotics is common and alarming

The material in this chapter is based primarily on the findings of research conducted during 1974-1976 in a leprosy control scheme in Western Province, Kenya, where an attempt was being made to combine leprosy and tuberculosis services and to integrate them within the general health care delivery system. Team members were Iman Bijleveld, Titus J. K. Gateers, Carla I. Rissecuw, Jan G. J. M. Ruyssenaars, and Corlien M. Varkevisser. The study was made possible by grants from the Dutch Directorate for Technical Assistance, the Foundation for Scientific Research in the Tropics, the Netherlands Leprosy Relief Association and the Royal Tropical Institute, Amsterdam. References appear as well to similar research conducted simultaneously in neighboring Mwanza Region, Tanzania.

to observe, all the more so when these "wonder drugs" are given in an inadequate dose. At Kenyatta Hospital in Nairobi, to call attention to an extreme and yet not unrepresentative situation, open heart surgery is now available, although there are still rural areas urgently in need of dependable basic health services. In analogous fashion, expensive, illustrated color brochures have been distributed in Kenya advertising "antidepressants," while drugs and vaccines for some major infectious diseases are not readily available. Indeed, it is often not a matter of doing too much, as Illich would claim, but doing too much of the wrong things — spending money on research topics or health facilities of peripheral importance to public health rather than where it is needed. Misspending thus, not overspending. The pharmaceutical industry above all appears dictated by profit considerations, often to the detriment of public health (Ferguson, 1981). Emulation of Western medical models without consideration of the indigenous population's real health needs is criminally wasteful for developing countries with limited resources. Furthermore, there are numerous examples of medicalization (e.g., in mental disorders) in which longstanding traditional treatment may be every bit as good as what Westerners have to offer, or may, with minor modification, be improved until acceptable by modern standards.

In this chapter, however, overmedicalization will concern us less than modern medicine's shortcomings in dealing with health care needs in developing countries. We will describe shortcomings in leprosy control programs in East Africa that arise from a lack of rigor rather than from too much medical care (Varkevisser, 1977; Ruyssenaars, 1978; Bijleveld, 1978a and 1978b). Wrong or sporadic delivery of dapsone (DDS) to leprosy patients, for example, has created a drug resistance problem. This is a worldwide phenomenon, as was made clear at the XI International Leprosy Congress in Mexico City in 1978. In spite of the availability of dapsone, a cheap and effective drug, patients have seldom received appropriate amounts for long enough periods of time, and now in various parts of the world, dapsone has lost and continues to lose effectiveness. An underactivity of medical systems has been responsible, and this is not only of a technical nature. System failures that undermine staff motivation and consequently patient compliance, too, may culminate in the total breakdown of effective long-term care. Treatment that is not rigorous may actually prove countereffective.

Leprosy in East Africa is a persistent problem. The disease is caused by an acid-fast bacillus related to that causing tuberculosis. Effective treatment for leprosy, as for tuberculosis, is of recent origin (1940s). The long duration of leprosy treatment (three years to life long) raises organizational problems, especially in rural areas where medical services are still underdeveloped.

Accessible delivery points for treatment are necessary as well as cooperation and mutual understanding between patients and health worker. In many places in the world leprosy is still thought of as incurable; treatment of the disease therefore may need to begin with changing peoples' perceptions. All, including lower health staff, must become convinced that early reporting for treatment will prevent unnecessary suffering and will stop the spread of disease to others. In the discussion that follows, a number of essential features of a successful control program will be identified.

CASE FINDING

Estimation of the prevalence of leprosy and the proportion of patients actually receiving adequate care presents great difficulties. When survey data are available, it becomes possible to determine what proportion of the total case load has already been registered for treatment. This may be high — 80 percent in the Wanga locations of Western Province, Kenya, where leprosy treatment has been available since the early 1950s. Usually, however, survey statistics are less favorable. Most registered cases are self-reporting, but the early symptoms of the disease are not well understood. Swellings are a common feature of leprosy reactions, but many patients do not interpret them as part of their disease. In traditional patterns of thought, swellings go paired with witchcraft. To treat a leprosy reaction, therefore, a patient may visit a specialist in witchcraft.

Furthermore, leprosy is stigma; emergent patients fear that they will be made the object of discrimination as soon as their condition is made public. Attempts to avoid disclosure, the wish to keep one's secret, can postpone the date when a patient first reports to a leprosy clinic. Assuming certainty that the disorder is leprosy, new patients choose between two risks: do not go for treatment and risk physical deterioration or go for treatment and risk stigmatization. The first risk is often preferred. At the same time, stigma inhibits people in the vicinity of leprosy suspects from approaching them in order to persuade them to seek modern treatment. It is not merely bad "form" to talk with leprosy patients about their illness, it can even prove dangerous. Should a quarrel erupt, an exchange of blows even, then the giver of advice may be fearful of contracting leprosy; for it is commonly believed that leprosy patients who feel insulted gain revenge after death by passing on the disease.

The silence about the disease within which leprosy patients are condemned to live thus complicates the considerable difficulties of effective control. That the stigmatization that emergent patients fear turns out later to be far milder than their expectations had led them to believe, does not in any way prevent those early excessive fears from interfering with the decision to report quickly for modern treatment. *Successful leprosy control must therefore begin with creating a climate within which leprosy "suspects" need not hesitate to consult medical opinion.* This entails reduction of public fear of leprosy through both adequate health education and dependable medical services (Bijleveld, 1977, 1978).

COMPLIANCE

Even when case-finding has been rather successful, only a small proportion of patients can be considered to be "under control," which refers to whether a patient has attended at least 75 percent of his scheduled clinic visits or has been discharged as cured. Neither in Western Province nor in Mwanza Region, Tanzania, were more than 30 percent of known patients under control. Research has taught us convincingly that it is the quality of leprosy services in the field that ultimately determines the consistency of patient attendance and compliance. Originally, we had been asked to investigate what were the social and cultural factors interfering with regular patient attendance at the clinics of the West Kenya Leprosy Control Scheme. We discovered, however, that formulation of the problem in this manner was misleading, for it implied that in looking for our explanation of poor attendance we should concentrate exclusively on *patient* behavior, lodging responsibility squarely on the patients' own shoulders. In areas of Western Province, having rather homogeneous populations, attendance rates at leprosy clinics had been recorded that varied exceedingly. Some clinics boasted almost optimal regularity of attendance. Attendance at others was deplorable. Clearly social and cultural factors by themselves could not account for the gaping difference.

To test the hypothesis that attendance was in large part a function of the job performance of the health worker at the base, we chose to study two samples of patients: (1) patients registered at clinics operated by a man who performed his responsibilities almost flawlessly and (2) patients who were to attend clinics of a man whose dedication to his work left much to be desired. The samples did not differ from each other in respect to age or sex distribution, nor in their representation of various grades of disability. Thus, all other factors being roughly equivalent, we could isolate the quality of services rendered and examine its impact on patient response.

Results demonstrated that when medical service is *regular* and when leprosy patients meet with *respect* and receive some degree of personal *attention*, they turned up for treatment punctually, there was virtually no defaulter "problem," and at home, independent of medical supervision, they faithfully swallowed their dapsone on schedule. (Urinalysis established the superiority of the dapsone intake-behavior of the "good" fieldworker's patients compared with regular attenders in Tanzania, Mali, and Ethiopia [Huikeshoven, 1978].)

Dissatisfaction with the job performance of medical personnel but also dissatisfaction with the speed of their own apparent recovery may lead patients to "shop around." They may consult traditional doctors — herbalists as well as diviners — who, although they have lost their health care monopoly still remain active. This is an established health-care-seeking pattern of behavior for the sick in Western Province: you keep looking until you find the doctor who achieves the best demonstration/effect of his abilities. Modern medicine can cure leprosy, but in the majority of cases progress with dapsone is anything but dramatic. It is gradual and sometimes barely perceptible. At some point during long years of modern leprosy treatment a patient may well turn to a traditional medical figure in hopes of rapid improvement. Such desertion is especially likely should a patient's condition appear to take a sudden turn for the worse while taking dapsone, for example, should one enter into "reaction" (i.e., suffer from complications of the disease that, however, one may fail to associate with leprosy).

Traditional treatment frequently involved and still involves a close bond between healer and patient. For some illnesses patients might even live in the compound of the doctor, a pseudokinship relation would develop, and the doctor would be addressed as "father." Consider the contrast offered by modern medical care: up to 300 patients a day waiting in line for a brief consultation, with health staff finding themselves busy in a sort of mass medical assembly line. It is often objected that whereas Western medicine reduces patients to symptoms, to parts of the body needing treatment, or to interesting specimens, traditional treatment remains personal. Again, overmedicalization is not the problem, but rather deficient relations between health staff and patients. In this respect it would seem that traditional treatment has something of value to teach.

Health workers are often not committed to service. They may be working at the only available job. In Western Province jobs are scarce: those who leave school who may once have had high ambitions now are eager to settle for any salaried employment. Motivation is important to job performance of any description, but especially in health care work. The training many receive, moreover is a problem in its own right. It does little to help new health workers develop useful attitudes toward the work they are to do. Time and again we witnessed health workers acting in harsh, *authoritarian* fashion toward patients – they were haughty; they were the "employed," the "educated" – and patients were "somehow ignorant" people from "the bush." "I am not the one who is sick," one leprosy fieldworker liked to remind the patients, "You're the ones to have to struggle for treatment. Or do you pay for this free government medicine?" Leprosy patients are to some degree fortunate in that they know what the medicine they receive is for. Commonly, patients at health centers are given medicine but no explanation of what is wrong with them. No questions are welcome.

Health workers at the base often find themselves in a "halfway" situation. They have recently emerged from rural, illiterate, traditional backgrounds and have entered into the process of modernization. Their roots have not yet been wrenched free of the past; their schooling, however, has introduced new values and new codes of behavior. Such "marginal" figures, people in transition, are prone to look down at their own background, at people who are like they were a short time ago. This helps account for the aloofness and the mockery patients encounter at health centers. And it helps account for why health staff pretend to be ignorant of traditional ideas and practices concerning the diseases they are called on to treat. This is highly unfortunate. An essential part of leprosy control is health education. To keep leprosy patients regularly on treatment it is necessary to inform them about their disease in ways that they can understand and accept. However, any health education that ignores traditional ideas about leprosy and any attempts to talk about leprosy as if a patient's head is empty and not filled with ideas common in the community will surely fail. Listening to a patient and sharing the traditional outlook in order to be able to present "modern" ways of thinking that will make sense is where health education should begin.

TREATMENT POLICY

Self-evidently, the kind of relations established between health staff and leprosy patients will depend largely on national policy guidelines and how they are applied in reality.

As long as no effective medicines were available, policy dictated the isolation of leprosy patients. Some have claimed that compulsory isolation (for tuberculosis) was an example of self-aggrandizement of bacteriologist-physicians (see Chapter 15). But long before the leprosy bacillus had been identified, local custom in many places demanded the setting apart of leprosy patients. In Western Province, Kenya, for example, such patients ravaged by their disease were finally forced to live in solitary seclusion along the banks of a river. Yet, there are counter examples, too, as in Northern Nigeria where leprosy patients were not driven out of their communities but carried on as usual with little or no stigma. In general, however, we can say that national policies assigning leprosy patients to leprosaria reinforced prevailing local beliefs that the community had to act to protect itself by keeping a safe distance from patients.

The advent of therapy with dapsone and the accompanying policy decision to begin outpatient leprosy treatment demanded organizational adjustment and a radical change of attitude, not only from local communities but also from health staff. Once policy prescribed ambulant treatment for patients near their homes, special treatment centers had to be created for leprosy patients where rural health facilities for general treatment were not widely distributed. "Tree clinics" mushroomed in sites selected because of their convenient location (e.g., markets, church porches, well-known crossroads, trees that were landmarks). Here leprosy patients from the neighborhood convened to meet a health worker who traveled to them, bringing medication. In the late 1950s and early 1960s in eastern Africa, these health workers were usually "specialists" (i.e., those with primary school educations who with a few months of training in leprosy treatment and equipped with a simple medicine kit and bicycle penetrated the area around their rural posts), the monovalent forerunners of present polyvalent "primary health workers." Leprologists hoped that by organizing leprosy services along these lines they could, at minimal cost, bring leprosy under control within the boundaries of their schemes within 10 to 20 years.

These hopes were ill-founded. Much less progress was made than hoped with these specialized leprosy services. Consequently, in Kenya a decision was reached in the early 1970s to attempt to combine leprosy and tuberculosis services and to integrate them into the general health care delivery system. (The duration of tuberculosis treatment, one to two years, raises organization problems similar to those already discussed for leprosy.) Tanzania soon followed Kenya's example.

Our research revealed how both public and health staff reacted with reservations to such a shift in health care policy. The new policy was sound enough, but unfortunately its implementation was not always preceded by adequate preparation. Certain basic measures were not taken in time. Although the recommendations that follow are for improving leprosy and tuberculosis control in developing countries, they may also be instructive in other, broader contexts. We must be careful to avoid making assumptions about what is obvious, for it is the obvious that so often proves easy to overlook.

Before integrated leprosy and tuberculosis services are launched, accurate and detailed job descriptions for all staff involved in leprosy or tuberculosis activities must be drafted. A trial period for seeing whether in reality workers can handle their assigned tasks adequately is highly advisable. Introduction of a national program for leprosy and tuberculosis usually brings with it an increased workload for general staff; the extra tasks involved may seem especially heavy because of the fears and anxieties that surround these diseases. Only the Ministry of Health itself has enough authority to exact the level of cooperation needed, and then only through careful explanation and persuasion together with official directives. The pilot project in Western Province would have been spared considerable difficulty had official support been forthcoming during its early days.

Lines of authority should be clear to all parties concerned. Especially where separate leprosy schemes have existed previously (as in Kenya and Tanzania) confusion is likely after "integration" about who is to supervise whom. The position of expatriate doctors who continue in service after nationalization of voluntary agency schemes and the position of former leprosy/tuberculosis supervisors at district level need careful delineation within the general health care hierarchy. The destructiveness of the lack of supervision arising from authority conflicts was illustrated both in Western Province and in Mwanza Region during the difficult early days of "integration."

All staff involved in any way with leprosy and tuberculosis patients should be trained adequately for the work they must do. In places where separate services formerly existed, or where only a fraction of general health care staff ever dealt directly with the patients of these two diseases, general medical training more likely than not still skips anything but perfunctory mention of certain bare facts concerning leprosy or tuberculosis. Without revision of curriculae and the introduction of in-service leprosy and tuberculosis training, no combined, integrated leprosy and tuberculosis services can hope to succeed. This may be categorical but we feel it to be true. In Western Province the pilot integration project had no leverage it could use to introduce new subjects into the general medical training program. It organized local in-service training courses but could not train staff in sufficient numbers to prepare all within the province who were to assume new leprosy or tuberculosis tasks before the summary "implementation" of integration.

In Mwanza something of the reverse problem emerged: part of the general health care staff were trained for leprosy duties, but plans for integration were realized with such delay that retraining was necessary by the time actual leprosy patients were coming to them for treatment. Rapid turnover of medical staff in both areas (transfer after 1½ years is average), moreover, erodes the value of any local in-service training. Once integration has been achieved nationally, shifts of health personnel from one place to another will be less disruptive; yet we should not underestimate the value of continuity in the relations between staff and the leprosy or tuberculosis patient. When the personnel of a given treatment center have worked together sufficiently to constitute a team, the benefits for tuberculosis and leprosy control are undeniable.

The training provided to health workers involved in leprosy or tuberculosis control responsibilities should above all be practical. The health staff must not merely be overwhelmed with scientific facts. Understanding and assimilation of new information is essential to enable the health staff to communicate effectively with patients and healthy community members.

Continuous supervision and encouragement, as well as constructive criticism, is necessary above all during the early years of integration. Punctual, dependable visits by personnel from the district and regional level will help sustain workers at the base; the failure of supervisors to turn up on schedule will, on the other hand, undermine morale.

Medicines and additional equipment require systematic distribution. Shortages of basic drugs at treatment centers arose, in most instances that we observed, from poor planning rather than from lack of funds. Transportation, of course, can interfere with distribution but then planning as far as transportation was concerned also in many places left much to be desired. It would be folly to contemplate introducing an expensive multiple drug regimen for leprosy or tuberculosis given present deficiencies in the distribution of thiazides and dapsone to many peripheral health units. When poor organization inflicts drug resistance on patients, they are being victimized in a most grave, irresponsible fashion.

These observations on leprosy control in East Africa are perhaps characteristic of the imposition of Western-style medicine in a developing country, but the problems and the shortcomings of leprosy control in this setting hardly seem to represent *over*medicalization. Rather they are examples of an unprepared transfer of technology to an ancient problem in an ancient culture. Illich's tirade against dysfunctional medicalization is surely useful. The careful questioning of the benefits arising from any system that we usually take for granted will invariably alert us to dangers at the same time, dangers that might otherwise escape notice. In developing countries, however, rural health care has a long way to advance before its excesses will form a major concern for public welfare. Its deficiencies and how to remedy them still require most of our concern.

REFERENCES

Bijleveld, I. 1978a. *Leprosy Care: Patient's Expectations and Experiences.* Amsterdam: Royal Tropical Institute.

Bijleveld, I. 1978b. *Leprosy in the Three Wangas, Kenya: Stigma and Stigma Management.* Amsterdam: Royal Tropical Institute.

Fergusen, A. E. 1981. Commercial Pharmaceutical Medicine and Medicalization: A Case Study from El Salvador. *Culture Medicine and Psychiatry* 5:105-34.

Huikeshoven, H., and Bijleveld, I. 1978. Encouraging Results from DDS Urine Analysis among Registered Leprosy Patients in the Three Wangas, Kenya: An Exception That Challenges the Rule. *Leprosy Rev.* no. 49, pp. 47-52.

Illich, I. 1976. *Medical Nemesis: The Expropriation of Health.* New York: Pantheon.

Ruyssenaars, J. 1978. *Leprosy in Mwanza Region, Tanzania: Background for Integration into the Basic Health Services.* Amsterdam: Royal Tropical Institute.

Varkevisser, C. M.; Risseeuw, C.; and Bijleveld, I. 1977. *Integration of Combined Leprosy and Tuberculosis Services within the General Health Care Delivery System, Western Province, Kenya.* Amsterdam: Royal Tropical Institute.

PART V

The Interface between Western and Traditional Medicine

The beliefs, methods, and focus of Western medicine are different from those of traditional medicine. When they come into confrontation, the traditional forms are likely to be the losers in spite of great advantages they may offer culturally, psychologically, and economically. Western medical ideas may be used inappropriately, as in the case cited by Sangree in Chapter 18 in which the control of sleeping sickness was used as the rationale for destroying a sacred grove.

More commonly the Western model is revered as the only model to be emulated with recently trained health professionals despising or avoiding the potential contributions of traditional medical care as in the case in Tanzania described in Chapter 19 by McCusker in which newly trained medical graduates wish to suppress traditional practices.

In Chapter 20, Quick describes the mixed motivations and styles of World Health Organization committees and national medical planners in developing countries who work toward a fruitful amalgamation of Western and traditional practices. The risk that he perceives is that traditional medicine is inserted into and co-opted by Western models without retaining the great strengths of the deep cultural embeddedness of traditional models. Lasagna in Chapter 21 notes similar risks in the injudicious and uncritical promotion of either model whether in the use of drugs or strategies of health care. The best should be extracted from each model.

A consensus emerges that the skillful blending of Western and traditional models has much to offer: the Western model particularly in technical advances, and the traditional model particularly in holistic approaches intimately tied to the cultural and parochial needs of a community.

18

THE MISCARRIAGE OF
MODERN PUBLIC HEALTH POLICY:
Tribal Ritual and Mortality Rate
among Irigwe Priest Elders

Walter H. Sangree

In 1963-65 I carried out field research among the Irigwe and I was struck by a peculiar relationship between Irigwe social behavior and patterns of authority and the mortality rate. In 1970 I published an account of the relationship between sleeping sickness, ritual leadership, and Irigwe world view (Sangree, 1970). It appears that my formalization and publication of this relationship had unanticipated consequences — that is, consequences unanticipated by me, and of a very questionable nature for health care. First I shall summarize the nature of this relationship, and then I shall outline the unanticipated consequences of my making it known in a scholarly publication.

HEALTH AND THE AUTHORITY AND
BELIEF SYSTEMS IN IRIGWE

The tribal area of the agricultural Irigwe, just above the western escarpment of the Jos Plateau, is virtually denuded of forest except for several sacred groves that people are forbidden to enter except for ceremonial purposes. Irigwe is a segmentary society that lacks

I wish to thank Bre Goji for his assistance with this report. All statements of fact and interpretation are made on the basis of my own understanding and judgment, however. I also wish to express my appreciation to the National Science Foundation, which funded my research in Irigwe in 1963-65.

a traditional centralized political chieftaincy. The highest religious authority within the tribe is traditionally accorded to the ritual elders of two of the tribal subdivisions who are in charge of the sacred ritual that is held to be of supreme importance to the well-being of the tribe as a whole. It is believed that the forces controlled by this ritual bring life to the tribe, but only at the cost of frequent death to members of those subdivisions of the tribe controlling the ritual.

There are 25 tribal sections, and the ritual elders of two of the smallest sections tend ritual in the sacred groves. The ritual elders of these two sections not only regulate much of the ritual of the tribe as a whole but also effectively intermediate between other sections in cases of intersection disputes. Each of these sections is also ever on guard against the other section's usurpation of tribe-wide supremacy. The two largest but ritually unimportant sections formerly supplied most of the tribe's secular leadership for warfare and today provide leaders for the British-instituted tribal administration. The Irigwe justify the high regard in which the ritually powerful sections are held and also explain their small size by their belief that the forces controlled by these sections, while vital to the tribe, are very dangerous and often kill those families who handle them.

The ritual elders, and particularly the most senior ritual chief, of each section suffer from two sorts of stringent constraints on their behavior and their exercise of authority. First, the ritual chief and elders have a particular ritual and authority role ascribed to them by the position their section occupies in the ritual and authority structure of the tribe and they fear dire consequences for their section and all Irigwe if they fail to fulfill or if they overstep the limits of these traditional responsibilities. Whenever any part of the annual ritual cycle is mishandled, it is believed that calamity will follow – usually in the form of weather adverse to the appropriate seasonal activity – with disastrous results for the entire tribe. Thus, the conduct of every section's ritual chief and elders is very much the concern of every other section's ritual chief and elders.

The second kind of constraint on the behavior and authority particularly of the section ritual chief is his fear of illness and untimely death for himself if his actions displease the nature spirits and ancestors of his own section. Irigwe notions about disease are complex. A major factor in every individual's health is believed to be the favorable disposition of one's relatives and the spirits of the dead, particularly the spirits of one's agnates. The Irigwe believe that anger in the hearts of living agnates, or the vengeful spirit of a deceased relative, makes it difficult or impossible for a person to recover from injury or illness, even though a partial or primary cause for injury or illness is attributable to some other agent. In addition, the nature spirits frequenting the section shrines and sacred groves not only may bring tribe-wide natural disaster if their laws are violated but also are held generally to bring ill fortune and speedy death to those individuals who abuse them.

The dangers of dealing with the world of spirits was a theme I heard again and again from the earliest weeks of my field work in Irigwe. Lists of ritual elders who had become the ritual chiefs of their section only to die shortly thereafter, purportedly because they had bungled one or another ritual and had been killed by the spirits, were recited as evidence. Youths of senior lineages of each section start their apprenticeships under their respective ritual chiefs early in their teens so that they will be well trained and will not fear to assume office if they live long enough to fall heir to the position of ritual chief. Each section feels obliged to guard the esoterica of its ritual from outsiders, indeed from all except those men and youths within their own section who are serving as ritual apprentices, fearing death to the ritual leaders and/or natural disaster to the tribe if outsiders should learn the secret lore.

Although people were too circumspect to discuss the topic publicly, it was widely recognized that the two most senior sections that controlled and performed the bulk of ritual for the entire tribe had not grown in numbers as much over the generations as had many other sections. Indeed, each of these sections has less than one-sixth the population of the largest Irigwe section, and they are considerably below the average section size. I thought the small size of these two sections might be due primarily to segmentation and the accretion of dissident lineages to other sections, but I was unable to find any evidence that this happened more frequently with these two sections than with most other sections.

About three months before I concluded my research in Irigwe, I had the opportunity to visit the government archives in Kaduna and found a mimeographed report on a trypanosomiasis survey conducted in Irigwe in 1932 by a government medical officer (Moir, 1933). A remarkably thorough job, it included a complete census of the tribe, which then numbered around 13,000, followed by a medical examination of over 99 percent of the population for sleeping sickness. The diagnosed cases were reported as being relatively benign, probably seldom lethal in themselves, with most sufferers complaining only of an occasional headache. It was found that the incidence of sleeping sickness was over 12 percent for males living south of the River Ngell in Kwol District, less than 6 percent for males living north of the River Ngell in Miango District, and under 2 percent for females throughout both districts of the tribe. The report noted that these differences could probably be accounted for in part by women's exclusion from the sacred groves, which happened to be the principal areas of tsetse fly infestation, and by the greater involvement of men in tribal ritual held in these groves, almost all of which were located south of the River Ngell in Kwol District. The report concluded by asserting that sleeping sickness was directly and indirectly causing a reduction of population in Kwol District, whereas in Miango District it was having no such effect.

The medical officer did not collect the figures for the incidence of sleeping sickness by section membership. It therefore remains unknown how closely the incidence rate of sleeping sickness for each section correlated with its relative involvement in the tribal ritual held in sacred groves.

During my last weeks of research in Irigwe I found a number of people who vaguely remembered the survey and several who recalled that many people south of the River Ngell had been treated for sleeping sickness at Government and mission dispensaries. Also I learned that the British-appointed Administrative Chief of Kwol District, who was a member of a ritually minor section, had cut down most of the forest under his section's control, starting in the middle 1930s, in spite of the protests of ritual elders from his own and other sections; all my informants insisted, however, that he had done this simply to sell the timber and pocket the money. It is noteworthy that none of the principal ritual groves of the tribe, all of which are under the control of ritually more senior sections, were cut down.

I had some success in explaining the possible long-term effect of sleeping sickness to younger Irigwe. One younger mission-educated man from south of the River Ngell, who had not heard of the 1932 survey until I discussed it with him, responded by saying, "Oh, that's why they are beating us!" He was referring to the fact that Miango District, the portion of the tribe north of the Ngell, which with one exception consists of ritually junior sections, has increased markedly in population with each census for the past 40 years, while the population of Kwol District south of the Ngell has remained more or less static, even though there has been little migration in or out of either district.

I doubt if I fared as well as the British had in the 1930s in my efforts to explain the sleeping sickness situation to Irigwe ritual elders. I remember all too well discoursing in my limited Irigwe on how sleeping sickness contracted by young apprentices in the ritual groves might through the years have checked the growth in numbers of the ritually most active senior sections; then, feeling beaten by my listeners' skeptical gazes I would find myself ending up by agreeing with my discussants that "There is indeed a lot more to health, illness, and large families than flies in the woods." The Irigwe elders agreed that ritually senior sections had not been increasing in numbers, whereas junior sections had; but their basic premise as to the reason for this phenomenon made my explanation seem simple minded and amoral, if not immoral. The senior section elders on many public occasions proclaimed their pleasure with the growth in population of junior ritually minor sections such as Nadzie in Kwol District and all of the child division sections in Miango District. "We are glad they are increasing, for they are our children," they would say. They asserted that if their own sections were not so populous it was because foolish people break the ritual law and that it is always the "parents" (i.e., ritually senior sections) that suffer the most on such occasions. Also, Irigwe elders pointed out that larger sections caught more game, the heads of which were deposited in the section shrines, than did small sections; and since section spirits like to have many heads brought to their shrines, the sections with the largest game bags obtained the most help from their section spirits in prospering and increasing in numbers.

The reason that the largest but ritually minor sections should hold most of the administrative leadership roles today as in former times was deemed a matter of common sense by the Irigwe elders. Which sections, they asked, could better represent the Irigwe tribe as a whole, both today in dealing with the central government in Jos and formerly in dealing with enemy and alien tribes, than the leaders of large sections with relatively great reserves of manpower at their immediate disposal for clearing roads or paths nowadays and for dealing with the enemy in battle in former times? Also, they asked, what kind of man makes a good administrative chief today and made a good war chief formerly? Irigwe elders assured me on a number of occasions that the attributes that an effective ritual leader must possess, such as a sober and exemplary personal life and an abhorrence of witchcraft and of alien doctrines, are in direct contrast to those an administrative chief may find useful today and those a war chief needed in former generations when dealing with an enemy. Indeed, in leadership when sacred rituals are not involved it was pointed out that being a witch (*krotu*), and even professing foreign doctrines such as Christianity, may be very helpful.

The notion that ritual power is dangerous to the ritual practitioner, especially if misused, is widespread throughout the world. Less widespread is the belief that sacred ritual power has a tendency to weaken and sometimes kill its practitioners even if correctly used. Here the Irigwe would seem to have developed a belief more or less directly in response to their empirically correct perception that sections of their tribe most heavily involved in ritual are in a moribund state as compared with those not so involved. The Irigwe view that secular leadership is appropriate for ritually subordinate sections may also have arisen from their awareness that those sections in fact produced by far the greatest number of warriors and war leaders.

Finally, the view I asserted, with which I know most Irigwe elders do not agree and which certainly is by no means proved, is that the tsetse fly has played a significant role in the "separation of church and state," that is, in the separation of Irigwe sacred and secular leadership and also, indirectly, in the development of the Irigwe ideology of ritual power and disease that supports this separation.

THE BUREAUCRATIC USURPATION OF RESEARCH FINDINGS

A preliminary version of the findings I have just outlined was presented at the 1967 American Anthropological Association annual meetings. Two copies were sent to a former research assistant, who by that time was attached to the museum at Jos, 20 miles east of Irigwe. One copy was deposited in the Jos Museum library, where an effort is made to keep an up-to-date collection of papers and publications on all nearby tribal groups. The paper was also sent to a small number of other English-speaking Irigwe whom I thought might be interested; and they did not send me any negative or critical commentary. Reassured by this I went ahead with plans to have the paper published.

Meanwhile, a major engineering project was underway in the area, including a new dam, sluiceway, and water conduit for the electrical generating plant that was being rebuilt and enlarged at Kwol (The Kwol II Development Scheme), which borders Irigwe to the west. My former research assistant worked as paymaster for the construction company (Balfour Beatty, Ltd.) after finishing his employment with me and before entering the museum school at Jos. The construction company found that the most direct and economically feasible path for the new sluiceway, given the contours of the land, was right through the northern portion of Chinkye Forest. This forest is the largest of the Irigwe sacred groves, which, as I noted in my paper, are very likely to be tsetse fly infested. The construction company's plans to obtain the necessary right-of-way through the forest were bitterly opposed by traditionalist elements in the tribe, particularly the ritual elders of the two most senior sections. I assume they opposed the company's plans principally for two reasons: (1) they feared the vengeful actions of the sprites (*rewienci*) which, according to Irigwe tradition, inhabit and guard the forest; and (2) they believed that cutting down the woods would "damage" the sacred ritual (*adzio tede*) by which they regulated hunting and farming activities and assured seasonable weather and that the tribe would thereby be put in grave danger of suffering crop failure or perhaps a pestilence or some other major natural disaster.

During the two years that my former research assistant worked for Balfour Beatty, Ltd. (March 1966-March 1968), work proceeded on the construction of the dam, while presumably the Kwol II Development Scheme officials carried on negotiations to obtain the right-of-way for the sluice through Chinkye Forest; it was not until the middle of 1968, however, that the development scheme, through court action, finally acquired the right-of-way from the Irigwe tribe and forest clearing and sluiceway construction there actually began. Proponents of the development scheme, who were very likely working either for Balfour Beatty, Ltd., or for the development scheme, took a copy of my paper (presumably the one deposited in the library of the Jos Museum) to the court hearing and presented it as testimony of an "expert witness" to help nullify the traditionalist Irigwe arguments against cutting down any of the forest. They used my paper to make the point that, contrary to the claims of the ritual elders, the health and well-being of Irigwe tribal members would actually be better served, according to modern scientific knowledge, if part of Chinkye Forest were to be cut down than if it were all allowed to stand, because the presence of the disease-bearing tsetse fly would thereby be diminished.

My former research assistant sent me no news of any later efforts by health authorities, or any other group, to continue or follow through on efforts to control or eradicate sleeping sickness in the Irigwe region; thus, I must conclude that I unwittingly supplied "expert testimony" in a context that clearly was not related at all to the health needs of the locals and that probably had little if any positive spin-off effect on their health needs.

In October 1968, my former research assistant wrote me that Kweshi, the ritual chief of Nuhwie Section (*baeri Nuhwie*) had died the previous September. Since Nuhwie Section is one of the two ritually most senior sections in Irigwe, Kweshi had in fact been one of the two most powerful and respected ritual elders of the tribe. He had always been very cordial and fatherly toward me when I was in Irigwe, but he had told me that I could not expect him to make me privy to the details of Irigwe sacred ritual (*tede*) because his doing so might not only endanger his life mystically but also the well-being of the tribe as a whole. I knew that Kweshi was well into his 80s and had held the position of shrine keeper for nearly a decade, which demonstrated in Irigwe terms that he had had the necessary knowledge, diligence, and moral purity to keep the powerful mystical forces of his office from killing him. I also knew Irigwe hold the view that very old people may simply die from senility. Thus, in my next letter I asked my friend to extend my condolences to Kweshi's family; I also inquired about who had been appointed to be the next ritual chief, but I did not think to ask about the circumstances of Kweshi's death. It certainly never occurred to me that there might have been a connection between Kweshi's death and my paper on sleeping sickness. That relationship was to emerge from later information.

THE MISCARRIAGE OF MODERN PUBLIC HEALTH POLICY

In September 1968, after permission to put the sluiceway through northern Chinkye Forest had finally been granted, and presumably after the cutting down of the forest in the right-of-way had already begun, a ceremony was held at which shrine keepers and elders of all the Irigwe sections were said to be present. As a body they judged that Kweshi, as the ritual chief (*baeri*) of the two most senior tribal sections, was in effect responsible for cutting down the trees in the sluiceway right-of-way through Chinkye Forest, even though he had always opposed and fought against that action. The elders demanded that Kweshi acquire a he-goat on that very day to sacrifice I presume to appease enraged sprites' and forbears' spirits, and thereby protect the well-being of the tribe. Kweshi agreed to make the sacrifice, but he refused to do it on that occasion, saying he would pick his own time and occasion. The other shrine keepers and elders kept pressing to do it that day and warned him that he might not live to see the next sunrise if he delayed. Finally Kweshi, after nightfall, left the group to return to his home, parrying their shouted admonitions and threats of the other elders with his own assertions that he would perform the sacrifice at his own time. Kewshi never reached his home. The next morning they found his body by the pathway leading to his home. There was no evidence of "foul play" or animal attack.

The above account of Kweshi's death is hearsay, or more accurately, "gossip." My friend, who was ill at the time, said he heard the story from other Irigwe. I have no reason to doubt that Kweshi actually did die in September 1968. Regardless of whether his death occurred under the circumstances that accord with the gossip, the general acceptance of the gossipers' story suggests that the cutting down of a portion of Chinkye Forest probably weakened traditional Irigwe beliefs as little as, indeed perhaps less than, it may have lessened the incidence of sleeping sickness in the area.

I personally am left saddened and humbled, particularly by the story of Kweshi's death. My sense of humility and sadness is all the stronger because early in 1965 Kweshi, who was as sharp-witted as he was spunky, in the presence of a number of other people, gave me, as Irigwe say, a special "midday name" (*lo tene*) — that is a nickname to fit my social role and behavior as he perceived it.

The "midday name" Kweshi gave me was "rabbit." Irigwe are farmers and they know as well as we do that rabbits have long ears that hear everything and that they lope around, looking harmless but eating in other peoples' gardens. Being farmers and hunters they also share Mr. McGregor's view that rabbits are best either chased away or trapped and eaten.

It would appear that Kweshi in 1965 had a much better insight into the implications of my presence and work in Irigwe for the Irigwe than I had. Clearly the belief systems that support social structural arrangements may be as relevant to individuals' health and well-being as more strictly biological disease factors. When the two are as intimately intertwined as they were (are?) in Irigwe, however, one needs to exercise caution in even making this interrelationship public knowledge.

In this instance, the decision to invade a sacred grove was rationalized as helpful to the public health of the community. A medical excuse was found to support the building of a sluiceway. This is certainly not medicalization in the ordinary sense; rather it is an abuse of medical knowledge for peripheral goals.

REFERENCES

Moir, J. 1933. Report on Trypanosomiasis Survey of Kwall and Miango Districts, Plateau Province, October-December 1932. Mimeographed. On file in the Northern Region Government Archives, Kaduna, Nigeria.

Sangree, W. H. 1970. Tribal Ritual, Leadership, and the Mortality Rate in Irigwe, Northern Nigeria. *Southwest. J. Anthropol.* 26:32-39.

ADDITIONAL SOURCES

Muller, J-C., and Sangree, W. H. 1973. Irigwe and Rukuba Marriage: A Comparison. *Can. J. Afr. Stud.* 7:27-57.

Sangree, W. H. 1969. Going Home to Mother: Traditional Marriage among the Irigwe of Benue-Plateau State, Nigeria. *Am. Anthropologist* 71:1046-57.

_____ . 1971. La Gemellité et le Principe d'Ambiguïté. *L'Homme* 11:64-70.

_____ . 1972. Secondary Marriage and Tribal Solidarity in Irigwe, Nigeria. *Am. Anthropologist* 74:1234-43.

_____ . 1974a. The Dodo Cult and Secondary Marriage in Irigwe, Nigeria. *Ethnology* 13:261-78.

_____ . 1974b. Prescriptive Polygamy and Complementary Filiation among the Irigwe of Nigeria. *Man* 9:44-52.

_____ . 1974c. Youths as Elders and Infants as Ancestors: The Complementarity of Alternate Generations, both Living and Dead, in Tiriki, Kenya, and Irigwe, Nigeria. *Africa* 34:65-70. Reprinted in Newell, W., ed. 1976. *Ancestors.* Chicago: Aldine.

_____ . 1976. Dancers as Emissaries in Irigwe, Nigeria. *Dance Res. J.* 7:31-35.

_____ . 1977. Irigwe Shrine Houses (*Rebranyi*) and Irigwe Concepts of the Sacred (*Tede*). *Savanna* 6:105-117.

_____ . 1979. Le Sexisme chez les Irigwe, Nigeria: Ses Contraintes et ses Correlats Soci-culturels et Économiques. *Anthropologie et Sociétés* 3:147-79.

_____ . 1980. The Persistence of Polyandry in Irigwe, Nigeria. In Women with Many Husbands: Polyandrous Alliance and Marital Flexibility in Africa and Asia, ed. N. E. Levine and W. H. Sangree. *J. Comp. Family Stud.* 11:335-43.

19

ATTITUDES AND TRAINING OF HEALTH PROFESSIONALS IN TANZANIA

Jane McCusker

The study by Varkevisser and Bijleveld on tuberculosis and leprosy control programs in East Africa detailed in Chapter 17 has described some aspects of the organization and quality of services provided by these programs that may be contributing to the failure to control these chronic diseases. The attitudes and training of health professionals are not only important determinants of the quality of services but may also influence the allocation of resources with the health care sector and the translation of national health care policies into practice. In this chapter I would like to review some of the work that has been done (including my own) on the attitudes of health care professionals in Tanzania and to suggest some possible effects of these attitudes on the development of health care services and on the quality of care.

There has been considerable interest in the development of Tanzania's health care system to see whether the unique solutions being attempted there may be a possible model for other Third World countries. Chagula and Tarimo (1975) have described the development of Tanzania's present system of health care services in detail. Tanzania is one of the poorest countries in the world economically. Its patterns of disease reflect this poverty and general lack of effective preventive services: high infant and early childhood mortality and high incidence and prevalence of malnutrition and infectious and parasitic diseases.

When independence was attained in the early 1970s, the British colonial system had left the country a legacy of hospital-oriented, primarily curative health services. A report to the government by the Titmuss Committee concluded that the country's health services were in a critical condition and that priorities should be placed on development of basic health services in rural areas and on preventive programs (Titmuss et al., 1964). These priorities were reflected in the First Five-Year Development Plan, 1964-69. The Arusha Declaration of 1967 set forth Tanzania's sociopolitical policy and stressed state control and ownership of the major means of production and distribution, self-reliance, and rural development. Following this, the Second Five-Year Development Plan 1969-74 intensified attempts to bring health services to the rural areas through the development of rural health centers, each serving a catchment population of approximately 50,000 and with several satellite dispensaries situated in villages. The development of *ujamaa* villages stimulated the moving of the isolated rural population to village communities to facilitate cooperative activities and the provision of those facilities essential to development: schools, water supplies, and health services. This attempt to bring basic health services to a large percentage of the population has been largely successful. Estimates made in 1973 indicated that while only 25 percent of the population live within ten kilometers of a hospital, almost 80 percent of the population live within ten kilometers of some type of health care facility (Thomas and Mascarenhas, 1973).

To run this pyramidal system of health facilities new cadres of health professionals have been trained. The medical assistant, who undergoes a three-year training period after completing secondary education, runs the rural health center and is responsible for preventive and curative services for a catchment population, including the conduct of general outpatient clinics and of mobile health services that make regular visits to the villages and sparsely populated rural areas and the supervision of dispensaries. The rural medical aide, with three years of training following primary schooling, runs the dispensary. At the apex of the pyramid is the district medical officer, a physician who is responsible for the health services of a district, including the operation of a district hospital. A system of regional hospitals is also being established, and three national referral hospitals exist. Physicians are trained at the Faculty of Medicine of the University of Dar es Salaam and following graduation are bonded to work in the national health service for five years.

Unpublished results of attitude surveys that I conducted among first-, second-, and fifth-year medical students at the University of Dar es Salaam in 1973 and 1974 revealed discrepancies between student attitudes and the work that they were being trained to perform. A substantial percentage of the students felt that rural work was slow and dull, that it was hard because of the superstitious beliefs of the population, and that it would lead to a deterioration in professional standards. Many felt that more resources should be directed toward teaching hospitals rather than to district hospitals. The majority felt that the period of government bonding was too long and that most physicians should have the opportunity to be trained in a medical specialty. Very few reacted positively to the ideas that more time during medical school should be spent in villages, dealing with health problems there, or that medical students should work for a year in an *ujamaa* village before beginning medical school. About half felt that development studies were not relevant for medical students. Regarding attitudes to traditional doctors and medicine, most felt that at best they were not effective and a substantial minority felt that they should be eliminated. In short, the attitudes of many of these students were similar to those of most students trained in Western medical schools and conflict quite sharply with Tanzania's national development plans.

It is worthwhile noting that the method of selection of these students, on academic performance, is similar to that used in Western medical schools and not noted for its ability to produce physicians with a strong social conscience or desire to work in medically underserved areas. It is of course debatable whether this method of selection is appropriate for medical students, and whether academic and technical excellence should be placed above social desirability. It is unlikely, however, that the attitudes described above will produce a district medical officer who is either well adjusted to rural work or satisfied with the level of care he is able to provide with the often sorely inadequate technical facilities of the typical district hospital.

Some results of these attitudes can be seen in the frequently expressed desires of medical school faculty for the latest technical facilities and equipment and in their concern for internationally acceptable standards of training. These attitudes may also be responsible for the continued imbalance of spending in the health care sector, with a disproportionate share of the funds going for hospital-related costs. Gish (1973) has argued for the inappropriate-ness of this spending pattern, showing that hospital care is in practice accessible only to a minority of the population, notably those living in or near towns or cities. Although theoretically, a referral system exists from the district to the regional to the national referral hospitals, in practice it is the population in the local area that comprises the vast majority of those utilizing and taking advantage of the technically more expensive care at these referral hospitals.

Van Etten and Raikes (1975) have described their work on the status and attitudes of medical auxiliaries in Tanzania. They point out the higher status of hospital-based auxiliaries (established during the colonial period to assist the physician) compared with auxiliaries in rural work, which is still reflected in differences in salary scales. They conclude that medical auxiliaries consider themselves as part of the clinical hierarchy and aspire to professional status.

Studies of the attitudes of medical auxiliary students revealed a predominant view of the rural population as ignorant and super-stitious (Van Etten and Raikes, 1975). The students tended to view rural people as extremely dependent on others and defined their own role in rural communities as one of expert and instructor. These attitudes are similar to some of those described in medical student studies and seem in keeping with the professional aspirations of the auxiliaries. In view of these observations it is ironic that one of the advantages frequently given for using auxiliaries is that the auxiliary is culturally and socially close to the people being served and has a good understanding of their problems (Flahault, 1973).

Other studies reported by Van Etten and Raikes (1975) indicate the existence of a set of attitudes and behaviors that run contrary to the principles of rural development strategy as being implemented by the Tanzanian government. They describe a "rural elite" composed of government staff involved in various village develop-ment programs, including health services, who are characterized by "frequent social contacts with one another, their identification with the richer farmers and their infrequent interaction with the poorer ones."

The intended role of the medical assistant, which was to provide both preventive and curative services, has not been effectively put into practice. My discussions with people involved in medical assis-tant training have led to the conclusion that a high priority in training is to persuade the medical assistant to think of the catchment population as a whole and to identify its special needs. The usual pattern seems to be for the medical assistant to become inundated by the heavy load of clinical problems that is confronted daily and to do little or no preventive or community work.

It is, as usual, easier to describe the problems than to prescribe solutions. Many members of the teaching staff both at the Faculty of Medicine and at medical auxiliary training centers in Tanzania are aware of these problems and have been and continue to be actively seeking solutions. It is probably true that health professional training should be realistic about the conditions of future work of the trainees and as far as possible should train them in settings that approach their future work situations. The Faculty of Medicine indeed rotates its students through the rural health center at Kibaha, near Dar es Salaam, and through the Bagamoyo District Hospital as part of their course in community health. However, most of their clinical training is still carried out at the University hospital, Muhimbili Medical Center, where conditions are far from typical of a district or even a regional hospital.

In 1974, the Ministry of Health made the decision to provide postgraduate specialty training in Tanzania for the limited number of specialists the country needs. The previous practice had been to send physicians abroad for specialty training. The training received was almost unavoidably inappropriate for Tanzania, and instead of providing these physicians with practical skills it taught them to rely on methods and technology that would not be available when they returned home. All too many postponed their return to Tanzania for several years or indefinitely, and many of those who returned became understandably frustrated and depressed with local conditions.

Another possible solution may be to lay greater stress on the teaching of medical sociology and social anthropology in medical school and in the training of medical auxiliaries. Leeson (1974) has referred to some difficulties in adopting this approach in Zambia. Although the Faculty of Medicine in Dar es Salaam does provide a basic course in medical sociology to first-year medical students, the message might be more effective if it were also incorporated into the clinical rotations.

The preceding account would suggest that the way that Tanzanian health care professionals define their role does not differ markedly from that in many other countries, including other African countries. This role definition seems to affect not only physicians, as might be expected, but also may extend down to the "front-line" medical auxiliaries. In view of national goals and priorities, this role definition is in conflict with the officially accepted view and may have dysfunctional effects for the health care professional and for the health service system as a whole.

REFERENCES

Chagula, W. K., and Tarimo, E. 1975. Meeting Basic Health Needs in Tanzania. In *Health by the People*, ed. K. W. Newell. Geneva: World Health Organization.

Flahault, D. 1973. The Training of Front Line Health Personnel — A Crucial Factor in Development. *WHO Chron.* 27:236-41.

Gish, O. 1973. Resource Allocation, Equality of Access and Health. *Int. J. Health Services* 3:399-412.

Leeson, J. 1974. Social Science and Health Policy in Preindustrial Society. *Int. J. Health Services* 4:429-40.

Thomas, I. D., and Mascarenhas, A. C. 1973. Health Facilities and Population in Tanzania. Research papers nos. 21.1 and 21.2. Bureau of Resource Assessment and Land Use Planning, University of Dar es Salaam.

Titmuss, R. M., et al. 1964. *The Health Services of Tanganyika: A Report to the Government*. London: Pitman Medical.

Van Etten, G. M., and Raikes, A. M. 1975. Training for Rural Health in Tanzania. *Soc. Sci. Med.* 9:89-92.

20

INTEGRATION OR CO-OPTATION:
Bringing Traditional Medicinal Plants into Public Health Programs

Jonathan Quick

Although traditional and indigenous systems of medicine have existed for millennia and anthropologists and medical historians have studied these systems for decades, serious interest in traditional medicine at the level of international health agencies such as those within the United Nations did not arise until the early 1970s. Within this decade, the World Health Organization (WHO), the United Nations Industrial Development Organization (UNIDO), and the United Nations Children's Fund (UNICEF) have all initiated projects to promote the use of traditional practitioners and traditional therapies. Among these agencies, the broadest and most active role is probably being played by WHO.

The World Health Organization is one of the focal points in what may be the largest international professional infrastructure: the allopathic medical profession. As such, WHO's involvement in the area of traditional medicine is likely to have a profound

---

This discussion is based on observations made by the author during recent visits to Peru, Costa Rica, Guatemala, Norway, Tanzania, Sri Lanka, Malaysia, and Papua New Guinea; on discussions with WHO officials in Geneva, Switzerland and at country offices; and on the cited published reports on traditional medicine.

impact on the future of indigenous and traditional medical practitioners and practices.

The purposes of this discussion are neither to applaud nor condemn WHO efforts. Instead, I wish to review briefly the history of WHO's interest in traditional medicine and to raise the concern that the motivations and content of current efforts to develop traditional medicine risk a reinforcement of the trend toward the imposition of the biomedical model of health care into the lives of tribal people and co-optation of traditional medicine by government programs.

Although WHO programs have interacted with traditional medical systems at the local level for many years, WHO traces its formal interest in traditional medicine to a meeting on the training, utilization, and study of traditional birth attendants held in 1972 at WHO headquarters (Bannerman, 1977; WHO, 1978a). During the next four years, the interest in traditional and indigenous medicine expanded and diversified. A 1974 UNICEF/WHO cooperative review of alternative approaches to satisfying basic health needs in developing countries supported the concept that practitioners of traditional medicine should be trained for primary health care services (Djukanovic and Mach, 1975). This concept was endorsed by the WHO Executive Board in 1975.

Activity in 1976 was highlighted by technical discussions by the Regional Committee for Africa on the role of traditional medicine in the development of health services (Bannerman, 1977) and by the formation of a WHO working group on traditional medicine. One outcome of this group's activities was an international meeting of experts in late 1977 that produced a monograph in the WHO Technical Report Series arguing for the "radical development and promotion of traditional medicine" (WHO, 1978a). The monograph outlined recommendations for an action program based to a large extent on the goal of integrating traditional and modern medicine in public health services. The views of this working group had received the popular support of WHO member states at the 1977 World Health Assembly, during which a resolution on training and research in traditional medicine was passed by acclamation. Most recently, at the 1978 World Health Assembly, the topic of traditional medicine was included in special technical discussions and was again vigorously supported by resolution (WHO, 1978c).

Thus the interest in traditional medicine represents a relatively recent movement and one that has rapidly gained momentum. This rapid rise in interest in traditional medicine raises two important questions. First, is the movement mostly rhetoric with little action? And second, what are the motivations behind the movement?

With regard to the first question, it can be pointed out that WHO is already in the process of collecting information on the names, descriptions, and uses of several thousand medicinal plants (Regional Office for the Western Pacific, 1977) and has begun collecting available literature on safety and efficacy evaluations of traditional medicines (WHO, 1976). A WHO Special Program in Human Reproduction is investigating the use of indigenous plants for fertility control in research centers located in six countries. The Working Group on Traditional Medicine is also focusing its attention on possible uses of traditional medicinal plants in treating drug dependence, cancer, rheumatoid arthritis, and the six endemic tropical diseases under study by the WHO Special Programme for Research and Training in Tropical Diseases (WHO, 1978a).

The motivations behind the WHO movement are undoubtedly manifold, but four stand out. The first is the perceived compatibility of traditional medicine with current efforts to promote primary care. After many years of encouraging targeted disease control programs, WHO has embraced the concept of primary care. It has devoted its efforts during the past several years to helping member states to develop integrated, holistic health services that are based on total community needs. The support of the local population, on which effective primary care programs depend, may be more easily obtained if government health programs are able to integrate local traditional medical practice with the modern health practices.

A second reason for pursuing the development of traditional medicine is the consistency of traditional medicine with the concept of "appropriate technology." There is a growing realization that modern technology is not necessarily well-suited to the needs of poor, small, and often unsophisticated communities in developing countries. The term "appropriate technology" is now widely used to denote the attempt to adapt modern technology to the needs of developing countries and, even more importantly, to exploit and to improve on those technologies that already exist and function effectively in developing countries.

A third factor in the growing popularity of traditional medicine, and one related to the issue of appropriate technology, is that of growing Third World nationalism and increasing effort to develop pride in indigenous resources and achievements. The growing number of Third World health professionals serving in WHO undoubtedly reinforces this influence.

Finally, the most frequently and emphatically stated reason for pursuing the development of traditional medicine is the very pragmatic realization that incorporating the already numerous traditional practitioners and exploiting available herbal remedies are necessary in order to achieve WHO's ambitious goal of "health care for all by the year 2000." Today the majority of the developing world's population does not have ready access to modern medical practitioners. This situation is not likely to change rapidly. A similar situation exists with regard to the availability of modern medicines. It is hoped that by encouraging the use of effective herbal remedies, the need for Western pharmaceuticals and the high cost of supplying medicines can be reduced. This view is expressed most clearly by Dr. Johnson-Romauld of Togo who, as chairman of the 1978 World Health Assembly Technical Discussions, concluded the session saying,

> To sum up on traditional medicine, I feel that it is the very shortage of modern medicaments in developing countries that provides one of the most cogent arguments for looking more closely at the resources offered by the traditional medicine of each country.

In one sense, the promotion of traditional medicine is an effort to redefine enough practitioners and therapies back into the realm of the officially acceptable in order to accomplish the task of providing "health for all by the year 2000." The interest in traditional medicine is expressed primarily as a desire to achieve the integration of traditional and modern medicine in public health programs. It is not completely clear what the term "integration" implies in this context. To determine what is intended, it may help to look more carefully at WHO's stated concepts of traditional medicine.

The WHO Regional Committee for Africa's 1976 technical discussion on traditional medicine defined traditional medicine as,

> the sum total of all the knowledge and practices, whether explicable or not, used in diagnosis, prevention and elimination of physical, mental or social imbalance and relying exclusively on practical experience and observation handed down from generation to generation, whether verbally or in writing. (AFRO, 1976)

The 1978 Technical Report Series Number 622 on traditional medicine emphasized the unique aspects of traditional medicine, stating that this form of care "has certain advantages over imported systems of medicine in any setting because, as an integral part of the people's culture, it is particularly effective in solving certain cultural health problems" (WHO, 1978a, p. 13).

The ideal relationship between traditional and modern medicine is described in the Background Document for Technical Discussions held in March 1978:

> Modern and traditional medicine should not compete with each other, because both are valuable national health assets. The former is based on the development of science and technology and the latter is based on national cultural values accumulated by the people over a long period of time. (WHO, 1978b, p. 32)

Thus, traditional medicine is characterized by its being based in the local culture and by its being derived from practical experience. It is differentiated from modern medicine, which is based on scientific discovery and on modern technology. Traditional medicine is described in positive, approving terms, and integration with modern medicine is encouraged. Despite this attitude, it would appear that the framework for integration is that of the biomedical model of inquiry and organization, which favors modern medicine. The previously mentioned 1978 Technical Report observes that, "effective integration . . . entails a synthesis of the merits of both the traditional and the . . . modern systems of medicine *through the application of modern scientific knowledge and techniques*" (Emphasis added) (WHO, 1978a, p. 16).

Integration of traditional *and* modern medicine appears to be interpreted as integration of traditional *into* modern medicine. Looking again at the 1978 Technical Report, "The Guidelines for Integrating Traditional Medicine into Primary Health Care" include as their first two points the following: (1) giving recognition to traditional practitioners and incorporating them into community development programs and (2) retraining traditional practitioners for appropriate use in primary care (WHO, 1978a, p. 14).

There is an ambivalence between the view that asserts that traditional medicine is a system that has certain inherent advantages and the view that its practitioners need retraining and must be incorporated into the community development programs. This ambivalence may stem in part from the political diversity of WHO. The effect of this diversity is illustrated by the interactions over the resolution on traditional medicinal plants at the 1978 World Health Assembly (WHO, 1978c).

The draft resolution, proposed primarily by developing countries speaks of the "ever-increasing importance of medicinal plants" and advocates for setting some international specifications for "crude drugs" and "simple preparations." Its interest is in "improving the use of medicinal plants." This version of the resolution appears to have been perceived by some countries as onerously positive and permissive with regard to traditional medicine. The final version (Table II) in which the United States, Switzerland, the German Democratic Republic, and other new countries participated in redrafting, is strikingly different.

The text of the final draft discusses the study of traditional herbal plants in a way that pulls them from their cultural and social setting and applies the same criteria to them as are applied to the study of drugs. The resolution advocates international standards for identity, purity, and strength; it encourages the development of directions so that medicinal plants can be used by "various levels of health workers" (presumably those already engaged in public health programs based on modern medicine), and it proposes the development of information that would allow mass production of medicinal plants. This approach is reminiscent of the efforts that the pharmaceutical industry is said to have made during the late 1950s to discover new active substances from extraction of ingredients from traditional medicinal plants.

Thus, there is a great deal of momentum favoring the exploration and development of traditional medicine, but the form of this exploration and development is largely the biomedical model of modern medicine. In social science research it is sometimes said that results are determined more by the way in which the questions are asked than by the underlying reality. Applying this to the current WHO activities, it can be argued that the framework that WHO is using may sharply limit the scope of the results. Probably the most important limitation is created by removing the traditional practices from their cultural setting for study and development purposes.

In light of the basic biomedical flavor of the international approach to traditional medicine, it is reasonable to ask whether

TABLE II
First Draft and Final Official Version of World Health Assembly Resolution 31.33: Drug Policies and Management: MEDICINAL PLANTS*

Draft Resolution on medicinal plants sponsored by the delegations of Italy, Malaysia, Rwanda, Togo and Viet Nam:	*Final Official Version of Resolution sponsored by the delegations of Ghana, Italy, Malaysia, Romania, German Democratic Republic, Rwanda, Sri Lanka, Switzerland, Togo, United States and Viet Nam:*
The Thirty-first World Health Assembly;	The Thirty-first World Health Assembly;
Having considered the *ever-increasing importance* of medicinal plants in health care, particularly in developing countries;	Recognizing the *importance* of medicinal plants in the health care systems in many developing countries;
	Noting the increasing awareness of governments and the scientific and medical communities of this matter;
	Considering that these plants contain substances which may be of therapeutic value but which may also possibly show potential toxicity when improperly used;
	Realizing that the use of medicinal plants is likely to continue in many countries;
Noting with satisfaction that WHO has already organized meetings on medicinal plants in the regions;	*Noting with interest* the efforts of the World Health Organization to deal with this matter;

260

REQUESTS the Director-General:

(1) to compile an inventory of medicinal plants used in the different countries and to standardize botanical nomenclature for the ones most widely used;

(2) to complete and update periodically a therapeutic classification of medicinal plants, related to the therapeutic classification of all drugs;

(3) *to review the available scientific data relating to the efficacy of medicinal plants in the treatment of specific conditions and diseases*, and make available, in summary form, the results of the review;

(4) to coordinate efforts of the Member States to:

— develop and *apply scientific criteria and methods for proof of safety and efficacy* of medicinal plant products, especially galenical preparations;

REQUESTS the Director-General:

(1) to compile a list of medicinal plants used in the different countries and to establish international nomenclature for the ones most widely used;

(2) to establish *international specifications for* the most widely used *crude drugs* and *simple preparations* thereof;

— develop *international standards and specifications of identity, purity and strength* for medicinal plant products, especially galenical preparations and *manufacturing practices* to achieve these ends;

(continued)

TABLE II, continued

Draft Resolution (continued)	Final Official Version (continued)
(3) to collaborate with countries desirous of *improving the use* of medicinal plants and/or their derivatives;	— develop *methods for safe and effective use* of medicinal plant products, especially galenical preparations, including *labelling* containing adequate *directions for use and criteria for use* for prescription by various levels of health workers;
(4) to coordinate regional efforts in the screening, scientific evaluation and better use of medicinal plants;	
(5) to disseminate information on methods of scientific evaluation of vegetable drugs;	(5) to disseminate information on these matters among the Member States;
(6) to designate regional research centers for the study of medicinal plants;	(6) to designate regional research and training centers for the study of medicinal plants;
(7) to ensure collaboration with other United Nations specialized agencies;	
(8) to report on the subject to a subsequent Health Assembly.	(7) to report on the subject to a subsequent World Health Assembly.

262

*Emphasis added.

Source: WHO. 1978. Drug Policies and Management: Medicinal Plants. World Health Assembly Resolution 31.33. Geneva: World Health Organization.

the current efforts to promote traditional medicine will serve to legitimize the role of traditional practitioners in government programs and lead to greater use of their services or whether it will simply remove traditional remedies from their cultural context, systematically study them and then incorporate the most effective ones into the therapeutic armamentarium of modern medical practice. If the former occurs, then a true form of integration will have occurred. However, if the latter occurs then the traditional healers will lose much of their special power — they will have been pillaged of their potions — and the Western emphasis on the thera-peutic agent, rather than the entire therapeutic process, will be reinforced.

In summary, the purpose of this chapter is neither to promote nor argue against international involvement in the study of tradi-tional medicine. Instead, it is to offer the caution that this process, if pursued along a strictly biomedical framework, may lead to co-optation, rather than integration of traditional medicine. The current international efforts to promote traditional medicine consti-tute a process that is near its inception. Opportunities exist to influence this process and, therefore, it can be hoped that the point of view that recognizes the uniqueness and cultural foundation of traditional medicine will guide the process toward a real integration of traditional medicine and avert the co-optation of traditional medicine by modern medicine.

REFERENCES

AFRO. 1976. *African Traditional Medicine*. AFRO Technical Report Series, Number 1, pp. 3-4.

Bannerman, R. H. 1977. WHO's Programme in Traditional Medicine. *WHO Chron.* 31:427.

Djukanovic, V., and Mach, E. P., eds. 1975. *Alternative Approaches to Meeting Basic Health Needs in Developing Countries*. Geneva: World Health Organi-zation.

Johnson-Roumauld, F. 1978. Address by the General Chairman of the Technical Discussions at the Thirty-First World Health Assembly. Geneva: World Health Organization.

Regional Office for the Western Pacific. 1977. *Final Report: Seminar on the Use of Medicinal Plants in Health Care*. Manila: Regional Office for the Western Pacific, World Health Organization.

WHO. 1978a. *The Promotion and Development of Traditional Medicine: Report of a WHO Meeting.* Technical Report Series, Number 622. Geneva: World Health Organization.

WHO. 1978b. Background Document for Reference and Use at the Technical Discussion on "National Policies and Practices in Regard to Medicinal Products and Related International Problems." Thirty-First World Health Assembly. Geneva: World Health Organization.

WHO. 1978c. Drug Policies and Management: Medicinal Plants. World Health Assembly Resolution 31.33. Geneva: World Health Organization.

WHO. 1976. Selected Bibliography on Evaluation of Traditional Medicines for Safety and Efficacy. Unpublished Document OMH/76.3. Geneva: World Health Organization.

21

THE PROS AND CONS OF WESTERN MEDICALIZATION VERSUS TRADITIONAL MEDICINE

Louis Lasagna

In discussions about the health care systems of developing countries, the term "medicalization" invariably has a pejorative ring, matching the criticisms by Illichites or holistic enthusiasts against Western medicine as practiced in its native habitat.

Yet for some of the most fearsome medical problems afflicting the Third World, it is to "medicalization" that one must perforce look for salvation. Malaria, schistosomiasis, tuberculosis, and the dysenteries are not fertile ground for holistic or even traditional plant remedies. DDT spraying in Sri Lanka almost overnight added years to the average life span of the Ceylonese, and the ravages of malaria soon became all too evident again when the people of that island were convinced by well-meaning Western do-gooders that DDT in fat tissues or in lower animals and birds was a worse menace than malarial trophozoites.

Indeed, Third World politicians usually berate the West both for not searching assiduously enough for new remedies for tropical diseases and for charging too much for the Western drugs desired by Third World physicians and patients. By their complaints, such politicians are acknowledging the fact that modern drugs, like eyeglasses, false teeth, artificial limbs, and cardiac pacemakers, are not to be ignored simply because they are not "natural."

Not all of the wonders of modern technology are desirable or feasible for underdeveloped countries. If funds, personnel, or equipment are in short supply, a CAT scanner may be an unaffordable luxury. Even in Western societies, there are great discrepancies in the extent to which physicians use laboratory aids or medicines. The United Kingdom, for instance, has long utilized data obtainable directly by the physician from history-taking and physical examination to a greater extent than the more technologically dependent U. S. physicians. The number of medications prescribed for the average U. K. hospital patient is significantly less than that for U. S. patients, nor is there evidence that British and Scottish patients are any the worse because of these differences.

It must be pointed out, however, that traditional medicine does not *necessarily* rely less on "therapeutic agents" than on the "therapeutic process." From what I have seen in China (Lasagna, 1975) of both outpatient and inpatient medicine, many Chinese are as oriented to their traditional medicines or acupuncture as Westerners are to their modern medicines or machines. Furthermore, certain Oriental philosophies encompass a resigned attitude toward death and disease, with individuals being insignificant parts of the vastness of nature. In such cultures, traditional approaches may be less supportive of patients than Western ideas might be. In regard to plant sources of drugs, it is easy for both Westerners and non-Westerners to forget that 25 percent of the modern pharmacopeia is derived from plant sources. Hence modern medicine cannot be said to neglect the plant kingdom. Dramatic progress has been made in recent decades by "rediscovery" of a few folk plant remedies. In the case of reserpine, the Indian usage of *Rauwolfia* plants was right on target. For the *Vinca* alkaloids, however, their remarkable oncolytic properties were not guessed at in the primitive use of periwinkle tea, which was erroneously thought to be a folk remedy for diabetes mellitus.

The three major ways in which medicalization seems to be important are the following: (1) the replacement of indigenous systems by foreign systems, (2) the substitution of less appropriate diagnostic and therapeutic models for traditional ones, and (3) the neglect of folk remedies.

The first two phenomena can have either bad or good results for a society, depending on what one is talking about. For many infectious diseases, as already indicated, modern antibiotics cannot be bettered by old plant or animal remedies. For those few cancers that yield impressively to chemotherapy or irradiation, it is foolish to eschew the use of modern remedies. For reversion of life-threatening arrhythmias, lidocaine is hard to beat.

On the other hand, the neglect of traditional medical systems can have serious untoward effects. For one thing, people used to witch doctors and native healers may not even be willing to seek help from a shiny, aseptic modern Western dispensary. No medicine can help patients who do not enter the therapeutic tent.

But there is the further difficulty presented by reliance on a Western diagnostic taxonomy and therapeutic strategy that may be inappropriate and ineffective. The routine prescribing of minor tranquilizers to the patients of an overworked Western doctor may in many cases be the best that he or she can do, but only because such a doctor has limited time to spend with each patient, does not know enough about the social context of each patient's complaints, and is often not skillful about manipulating interpersonal variables even if he or she were to have insight into nonsomatic causal factors. But in a small village, none of these limitations may apply to the local healer, in which case the nonpharmacologic approach may stand an infinitely better chance of producing relief or even more lasting effects.

In any case, each country should look on its health care system in totality and within the framework of the society as a whole. Drugs cannot be divorced from the availability of doctors and hospitals, to say nothing of food, sanitation, and population growth. Changes in the health care system need to be planned in concert with other social changes. Short-term planning should be different from long-term planning.

The total costs of health care can be decreased by efficient use of drugs — by a diminution in the use of unneeded drugs and an increase in the use of important therapies. The same applies to other medical technologies. Elsewhere (Lasagna, 1979), I have argued that a rational policy toward national drug production and extranational drug purchases is needed by each country. Rhetoric and polemics are no substitutes for reality, and in the particular area of pharmacotherapeutics a collaboration between the West and the Third World could achieve significant benefits for the sick with a minimum of delay.

REFERENCES

Lasagna, L. 1975. Herbal Pharmacology and Medical Therapy in the People's Republic of China. *Ann. Intern. Med.* 83:877-93.

Lasagna, L. 1979. The Diseases and Drug Needs of the Third World. *J. Chron. Dis.* 32:413-14.

PART VI

On the Use and Abuse of Medicine: A Conclusion
Marten W. de Vries
Robert L. Berg
Mack Lipkin, Jr.

MEDICALIZATION

Medicalization, as noted by Harper in Chapter 8, is making something medical by annexing what is not illness into illness (Sedgwick, 1978). This is particularly problematic where disease definitions of behavior occur (Szasz, 1961). Medicalization marks a change in medicine's degree of involvement in psychological or social areas. In the West, it has become fashionable to criticize such expansion while ignoring the universality of change and growth in medical systems across cultures (Janzen, Chapter 1; Fabrega, Chapter 2; Kleinman, Chapter 4).

The medicalization critics argue that concerns that properly should be directed at "medical" problems are now misdirected at phenomena that are really not "medical." They assume that problems involving disease and illness are of a distinct and special nature and that ways of dealing with disease and illness should not be used as a basis for dealing with other type of problems.

Medicalization is used as a pejorative term to connote corruption, aggrandizement, and clumsy medical activity. We felt that the medicalization criticism, indicting all of medicine as one, was simplistic and polarizing. Medical systems are both used and abused. They partake of both the best and the worst in people. Lasch, in Chapter 3, while not blaming the medic, holds that in the West, the integration of medicine in society has had a pernicious effect.

Following the work of Reiff, Lasch suggests that medical authority has become internalized as an organizational concept in society. An overgeneralization of the therapeutic relationship has occurred. This includes inappropriate altruism extended even into adversarial domains such as the courts and leading to departure from a free choice model of relationships. Medicalization has changed the negotiation of justice among citizens to the management of the irrational, the sick, or the unconscious. This is the *triumph of the therapeutic* (Reiff, 1966).

In evaluating this issue, we wondered whether "medicalization" could serve as more than a critic's device. Our approach consisted of looking to current and historical medical care models, preindustrial and industrial health care systems, and cross-cultural health care projects for paradigms and guidelines. We also examined one illness, couvade, in detail, as a model. International health care projects working at the cultural interface between Western ("industrial") and traditional approaches proved helpful examples because they offer an opportunity for observing medical conflict and expansion.

PATIENT AND PHYSICIAN

The mandate to alleviate suffering, with therapeutic activities, is taken seriously by most patients and practitioners. The overready willingness of the healer to accept supervision of patient behavior, however, may lead to usurping responsibilities better left with the patient, as Illich (1976) and Lasch (Chapter 3) point out. This would not be possible, however, without the patient's acquiescence or active seeking of a dependent or sick role, including the aroused concern and support of the individual's family and social network. A patient's anxiety with life stresses might be viewed as better managed within the family, religious, or educational institutions, but when these stresses are accompanied by somatic complaints, the medical care system is likely to be sought out. The potentiality for medicalization, and indeed the origin of the dyadic relationship itself, springs from the human longing for someone to lean on who has (mystical) knowledge and powers. The invoking of the doctor-patient relationship releases one of the most powerful weapons in the healer's armamentarium. It accounts for much of the compliance with medical regimens and of the placebo effect of drugs, while bringing to the patient the support of a caring authority figure.

At a conscious level the patient may exploit the system as a malingerer, to avoid work, or for sick benefits. The healer/physician may consciously seek much of the power and income of the medical profession as well as the satisfaction derived from helping the sick and is unlikely to be aware of the extent to which his or her own inadequacies are compensated by the respect, awe, and affection received from patients, not that the healer/physician necessarily seeks to make the patient dependent.

The ritualization of medical care not only enhances the evident power of the healer; it formalizes the relationship between the patient and healer. Only annointed or licensed healers may perform the rituals, label, and intervene. Sacred places, groves (Poole, Chapter 5; Sangree, Chapter 18), and hospitals (Pfifferling, Chapter 13) are reserved for their use. Sacred drugs (Quick, Chapter 20) are essential and their origins or nature are often held secret. The incantations and medical expressions are generally incomprehensible to the patient. This sacred language helps to reserve for the healer the ultimate mysteries of the origin of disease.

In addition, healers charge fees, have essentially a separate code of ethics, and claim prognostic and predictive powers. Western medicine has become especially powerful in this regard with its capacity to control jobs, careers, knowledge, skills, technological attention, and facilities. This is concretely evidenced in the United States, where medical activities garner 9.6 percent of the gross national product — 248 billion dollars in 1980 (Richmond, 1981).

Because of its capacity to consume resources and the formidable alliance between patient and healer, medicine is bound to be mistrusted. The reasons range from concerns about potential exploitation of patients' weaknesses or abnormality to envy and a displacement of anger at helplessness to medicine. The attack on medicine is aimed in part at demystifying and exposing the irrational nature of healing rites and trusting.

MEDICINE, SOCIETY, AND THE PRIESTLY ROLE

Co-optation of the medical care system by the politically ambitious is as distasteful as abuse from within medicine. The guardian bureaucrats, however, are less easily monitored. Since earlier cultures they have evolved roles that sometimes overwhelm the patient-healer relationship. They defend their status and resist procedural changes except those that increase their influence. At the boundary of the system, the ambitious chiefs may be enthusiastic partners in co-optation by political entrepreneurs who would use the medical care system as bait for larger schemes, as Sangree shows in Nigerian public health policy (Chapter 18) and as Brown suggests in Bismarckian Germany (Chapter 15). At times, this is more a matter of arrogance than abuse. In the development of an international formulary, for example, lip service substituted for collegial assessment of tradi-tional herbs and medicine (Quick, Chapter 20). This is sometimes matched by the misguided aim of some Third World leaders to sport a modern and large formulary (Lasagna, Chapter 21). Facilitated by private industrial interests (Ferguson, 1981), this process has led to the complication of infectious disease treatments in Third World countries, with a secondary effect of devaluing traditional treatments.

Abuse and neglect of this sort need to be exposed; yet, in reality, they hardly represent the totality of medical activity and omit those conscientiously attempting to heal and plan.

What then renders the expansion of medicine so odious? One does not think that it is wrong for business to expand; that is indeed one of its functions. But one does not expect this from medicine.

Medicine in exchange for power pledges a constrained approach to others. Because of oaths and "internal" controls, it is invested with trust, authority, and power. Its motives are expected to be altruistic, its function, protective and disinterested. When personal or questionable motivations occur, they feel sinful.

Abraham Jacobi's view of the physician at the turn of the cen-tury (Davis, 1916) as a "chum of the old people, the intimate of confiding girlhood, the uncle and oracle of the kids" has been greatly eroded. Nostalgia for a benign parental figure in the physician remains. Cross-cultural studies, however, point out that healers (like parents) are also feared and suspected (Ngubani, 1977; Evans-Pritchard, 1937; Turner, 1968). The dual, good and evil, nature of medical activity is highlighted across cultures. The healing arena, whether the examining room or homestead, is ambivalently viewed by the patients it serves. Medical activity, then, takes place in a loaded emotional atmosphere and partakes of our symbolic and cognitive notions and confusions about ourselves and our neighbors.

Opinions about medical care range along personal, cultural, and political dimensions. For example, when medical expansion occurs in a New Guinea society, it is the society that regulates patient and population compliance to medical rules. Romanucci-Ross (Chapter 12) suggests that groups have a differential capacity to accomodate medical systems, which may change over time. Medical activity does not occur in a vacuum and in many ways is inseparable from other aspects of society.

The patient healer and bureaucrat are, likewise, interlocked in cultural orientations and expectations of behavior, detailed in the couvade example (Poole, Chapter 5; Lipkin and Lamb, Chapter 6). The motives for medical expansion from all parties are often suspect, but the process itself can be either positive (Ciaglia, Chapter 16), natural (Janzen, Chapter 1), or negative (Brown, Chapter 15; Lasch, Chapter 3), depending on the standards of evaluation brought to bear on the outcomes sought by client and medical personnel. Medicine is not, however, absolved of its shortcomings merely because it participates in societal trends or responds to individuals' needs.

THE CRITIQUE OF MEDICINE IN INDUSTRIAL SOCIETY

Medicine has participated in the trend of society to resort increasingly to technical approaches in solving its problems. Specialization and professionalization have led to a further split of social institutions from community life. These artificial cleavages in the social system have been the by-products of technological advancement and the rapid increase in social complexity. The daily activities of individuals and the texture of living and dying are often far removed from more general social themes and issues.

The medical system, then, has evolved to a relatively isolated social position. Since World War I, the family doctor has changed from a community resource to a restricted hospital-bound practitioner of modern technique (Stevens, 1971). One root of the critique of modern medicine is the complaint that the modern healer's isolated position limits the capacity to meet the needs of the suffering human. Patients often experience chagrin that medicine is working poorly at the level that they experience as they struggle with pain, illness, and the desire to get better.

In addition, overly high expectations of technological medicine by both the patient and practitioner have resulted in patients often experiencing health care as depersonalized and alienated from other aspects of life. Technologic transformations (Kunitz, 1974) have actually had the effect of demedicalizing some of the integrated social functions of the traditional healer's role described by ethnographers and historians in this volume. The new remoteness of clinical activity has fueled patient dissatisfaction.

One medium of this process is medical training (Pfifferling, Chapter 13; Schiffer, Chapter 14). Medical schools divorce doctors from the day-to-day world and dehumanize trainees. Medical education is embedded in the economics of care and research. A trainee's role models are highly rewarded for doing procedures and for molecular biological research. There is low reward for humanistic concerns. This, too, is reflected in the language of medicine. The dominant classification fails to deal with the majority of illness (Lipkin and Kupka, 1982). Medical students are then trained to use biological reductionistic action models, producing a "culture of practice" in which clinicians consider only narrow technical hypotheses and generally do not care to see the connection of these disease states to the lives of their patients. The failure to consider human issues is a constraint to healing.

Clinical medicine's focus has narrowed increasingly to the "patient problem" despite efforts by reformers and educators to broaden the physician's concerns to include the family and work setting (Lipkin and Kupka, 1982). The growth of technology as well as the fact that it is simply *easier* to deal with an individual than with a (wider) social setting exacerbates this process. As medicine moved into larger institutions like hospitals, in order to make more efficient use of increasingly expensive technology (Stevens, 1971) practitioners were moved from the neighborhoods in which their patients lived. In addition, the social spectrum from which physicians were recruited narrowed (Kunitz, 1974). This served to make them less aware of the range of social, economic, and cultural forces acting on what to them seemed an increasingly exotic patient population.

While the changes in technological medicine outlined above resulted in increasing remoteness of clinical activity from normal life, another movement appeared. This contained the notion that the individual is responsible for disease prevention (Knowles, 1977). One impetus for this movement was concern about medical cost inflation and evidence that showed that life-styles are implicated in the cause of disease or at least shift the disease spectra. When added to the "public health perspective" that curing diseases is more expensive than preventing them, this contention had the pernicious effect of focusing blame on the individual while deflecting attention from the social institutions within which individuals are embedded. The ideologic belief that individuals themselves are responsible for their own misfortunes, whether those misfortunes were poverty, poor education, or ill health, implies adjusting individuals to existing institutions not reforming those institutions to meet the needs of the individual and citizen and thereby improving their health. Technological medicine in its concentration on the individual has both been allowed to hide from and ignore the social context in which its patients live. Medicine may therefore be accused of supporting "unhealthy" systems.

This form of the medicalization criticism is a reaction not to overpreoccupation with health and illness (Fox, 1977), but rather a reaction to overly expensive, depersonalized care that shies away from environmental causes of illness and does not deal adequately with the anxieties that many feel about their general well-being.

Illich sees the industrial system as the root cause of medicalization. He undertakes an attack on professional health care hierarchies as part of a larger attack on industrialism. Illich believes that industrialization *per se* creates technologies that are inherently dehumanizing, serving to give control over the patient's body and decisions about how to manage the illness experience to those who manage the technology. He advocates a solution in which the lay public will regulate health care providers and in which the equivalent of barefoot doctors would provide the bulk of care.

The result would be to return control over death, dying, health, and disease to lay people who would be weaned from dependence on professionals, drugs, and technological efforts to deal with intrinsically human experiences that ought not to be delegated. Illich's hope for achieving health for all is to eliminate the iatrogenic diseases brought on by the medical establishment. If a person must suffer, then it is the individual's right to suffer alone, autonomously. Illich puts it, "Man's consciously-lived fragility, individuality and relatedness make the experience of pain, of sickness and of death an integral part of his life. The ability to cope with this trio autonomously is fundamental to his health" (1976, p. 272).

Clearly, there are limits to therapeutic care, owing to the limited capacity of the healer's knowledge, available resources, and the nature of illness and mortality. We also agree that close interaction of a population with its healers is necessary. A community voice in the medical activities in their midst is part of a useful primary care model.

While we agree with Illich's essential humanistic concern, his romantic view that suffering is noble, for example, from tuberculosis or cancer, without the best medical care options, is, we feel, ignorant or arrogant. Every known culture has a health system because people universally desire health and shun sickness. It is absurd and historically false to imagine that health would somehow appear when released from labeling and treating systems of modern medicine. Illich confuses the cure's side effects with the problem! Clinicians and the medical system are part of social reality. They must be dealt with, not wished away or attacked like an external enemy.

We advocate the appropriate use of technological medicine practiced with sociocultural skill by clinicians embedded in community life, using methods consonant both with scientific knowledge and local social and cultural realities and constraints.

UNDERACTIVITY AND ALTERNATIVITY IN MEDICAL CARE

Predominantly Western concerns about health care have been addressed in the medicalization critique, such as the appropriateness of labeling behavior as symptoms and the healer's isolation from the community. We have seen that as medicine addresses issues of total health and the quality of life, ideological conflicts develop. Medicine's role becomes muted and confused in the patient's eye, and its advice becomes competitive with other systems, religious and legal, that define humanity.

In spite of this problem, health needs have been relatively well cared for in the West. Westerners live close to the maximum extension of the human life span. They have the luxury of training their medical technology on the quality of life rather than on day-to-day concerns with survival.

In the developing world, the situation is quite different. There, basic health needs have often not been cared for and high morbidity and a truncated life span results from infectious diseases, poor sanitation, overpopulation, and malnutrition. In this setting, underactivity and unplanned medical activity are stressed by some individuals involved in evaluating and providing care. Bijleveld and Varkevisser (Chapter 17) state that we have offered both too much and too little: too many drugs, equipment, and training that are either too expensive or cover the needs of only a few and too little organizational support and evaluation of existing medical care. They illustrate how essential it is for the improvement of health to fit Western medical care to local circumstances. Expatriate and indigenous health authorities work at the top and very little at the bottom in the health care hierarchy, even in community health efforts. McCusker (Chapter 19) links the overreliance on technologic medicine to general modernizing trends in the developing nations. She demonstrates that the influence of Western biomedical orientations on East African health workers quickly led them to perceive traditional medicine as inadequate. This attitude directly interfered with patient care and compliance. The crucial role of the orientation, attitude, and skill of the primary health care workers in providing anything that resembles adequate treatment is highlighted (Berman, 1978).

In international health care we have often erred by not learning more about the context of medical care, by not offering more help in allocating the limited resources of developing countries, and by not respecting traditional healing health care systems. Western medicine, while generally viewed as a salvation to people plagued by infectious diseases, is also criticizable for unthinking approaches, creating markets, spreading religion, placating people for imperialistic expansion, and disrupting traditional health care strategies over which technological medicine has no advantage.

The activity of Western medicine in the less developed nations teaches us at least four things: (1) medical care must be planned and integrated carefully into its social contexts; (2) the epidemiology and type of illness as well as its course is an important guide to the depth of involvement of health care activities; (3) the patient populations' "agenda," health care seeking strategies, and cultural modes of compliance are key issues in successful medical endeavors; and (4) a focused *selective* health care strategy is essential.

The underserved populations of both the West and less developed nations, such as the chronically ill, disabled, and the poor, tend to have health problems that can be managed only through increased medical intervention. For instance, in the case of tuberculosis, an illness we know something about, both adequate preventive and long-term treatment are essential. Long-term treatment requires getting involved with the patients' lives and changing their life-styles. While the content of increased involvement is different between the more and less developed countries, the principles are the same. Changing Western life-styles, such as habits of overeating, drinking, smoking, and the lack of exercise, are similar to changing habits in developing countries, such as wearing shoes to prevent hookworm, using uncontaminated water supplies for drinking and cooking, and providing enough protein in the diet to prevent mal-nutrition. Approaches to prevention and to the long-term treatment of chronic disease require different and more involved approaches than those for the management of acute illness. Medicine's increased involvement derives in the care of chronic illness from the nature of the patient's problem. Medicalization of disabilities would indeed be a boon to the chronically ill (Ciaglia, Chapter 16). Sadly, we are just beginning to understand how to provide this sort of care.

Who does what in this increased involvement of medical care remains contested. In international medicine, the question is always asked as to what roles traditional healers, lay therapists, commun-ity workers, or indigenous personnel should play. There is no spe-cific answer without a specified context. In addition to contesting who does what in providing technological medical care is the question of the role of other potentially competitive therapeutic institutions. These alternative systems are most visible in the Third World, but in the West numerous options are also widely utilized, such as chiropractors (McCorkle, 1961), herbalists (Green, 1980), faith healers and spiritualists (Harwood, 1972), as well as holistic and homeopathic movements (Pellitier, 1979). Although these movements are often in ideologic and practical disagreement, their activities coexist with the formal system. In developing countries the presence of technological medical systems apparently does not constrain other pathways for healing available to a population (Green, 1980). Such self-adjusting social and individual processes as Alcoholics Anonymous in the West and drums of affliction in Africa develop beside the larger medical system (Janzen, Chapter 10). The presence of technological medicine need not co-opt or drive out other systems. In fact, imaginative use of Western and traditional systems by the patient population may even prove helpful in plan-ning (de Vries, 1981). From the patient's point of view, the central-ization and limiting of health care seeking strategies in a population is not warranted. Choosing between multiple health care options need not be a problem and may be beneficial (Romanucci-Ross, Chapter 12; Janzen, Chapter 1).

Finding the right fit between a population's orientation and Western health care strategies is a delicate process. Each has much to offer; the Western model, particularly offers technological advances. Traditional models offer holistic approaches intimately tied to the needs and style of the community. The process of seeking agreement in who does what in health care usually does not evolve smoothly. It requires negotiation, trial and error, and patience. Successful clinical care is not dissimilar in developing or developed countries. Good medical care requires the universals of concern and availability, community support, a belief that the cure works, and some integration of the treatment modality with the rest of the patient's life.

RIGHT KIND OF MEDICINE

We differ from the medicalization critics because of our data and analyses. Szasz (1961), Illich (1976), Carlson (1975), and others have concluded that modern medicine has intervened with its therapeutic machinery into other social domains. They argue that medicine has infringed on or co-opted the therapeutic capabilities of the community at large, of the family, and of the self-healing capacities of the individual. This view has not stood up to the data from the world sample presented here.

The studies here, of varied cultures, have depicted an integrated relationship between society and its medical system, which also characterized Western medicine until this century. This interconnectedness has generally been seen as desirable. From this perspective, Western medicine does not appear as an overwhelming usurper of domains. Rather it looks more like an isolated subsystem, distant from the society at large, exercising a meager taxonomy in a relatively narrow field of concern while highly vulnerable to co-optation.

We have, then, reversed the complaint. Medicine in its training procedures, clinical activities, and institutions is not too big or too pushy but too distant from the realities of day-to-day life and broader social concerns. Medicine is too unaware both of the impact of its clinical endeavors and of the multiple forces that shape the expression of illness. The couvade example illustrates how this actually distorts and limits diagnosis and treatment. The problem is one of too narrow a language, too small a set of hypotheses, and too narrow modes of inquiry and action. The issue is one of inappropriate investigation and treatment, not of political or social inappropriateness (Lipkin, Chapter 9).

One's stand on the issue of whether society is overmedicalized, undermedicalized or whatever is interwoven with one's political point of view. We suggest that the problem with medicine is not primarily *how much* medicine but rather *what kind*. The question, then, becomes what is the appropriate fit of a given type of medicine with a given population? The material presented here suggests that the context of clinical activity needs to be fully included in answering. Only the reality of patient and healer's lives and the epidemiology of their illness, in concert with available resources, can adequately guide medical action.

In clinical care, this argues for a patient-and-population-based perspective (Lipkin and Lybrand, 1982). This means that the patient, while central, is always viewed as embedded in life and social contexts. The development of clinical care strategies that more fully evaluate and include the context of patients' lives and the impact of their illness experience is easier to say than to achieve.

In planning, population based health care needs to be developed (Lipkin and Lybrand, 1982; White and Bullock, 1980). The clinical approach should then be carefully balanced with the needs of the person, the community served, and the medical system. The crucial data — missing in most clinical approaches and assessments — is knowledge about the priority of problems and the context of the healing interaction. The assumption that medicine is powerful enough to create its own context has led to much ineffective and arrogant medical activity and is false. The real social context of curing must be assessed both from the patient and the practitioner's point of view. It must then be *negotiated*.

The flaw in medical care lies in the *inattention* to the psychosocial phenomena on which medicine impinges and which impinge on it. Not having or using those data results in negative or inadequate clinical activities (Lipkin, Chapter 9), the co-opting of other systems (Lasch, Chapter 3), or lack of awareness of the control by external forces (Navarro, 1975).

Treatment, like illness, must be experienced in life. Medical care should not just be the application of technology. Western medicine and institutionally based medical training must focus on life and illness history and community contexts. It is our belief that if medical activities are part of community life, both patient and healer will benefit. Certain principles about medical and social systems, discussed in this volume, provide a means of reembedding medical care in day-to-day life and negotiating patient-based care. Medicine must pay closer attention to the properties of other systems such as the communities' own models for health and disease and their pattern and strategies for seeking health care, including alternative and competitive approaches. Structures of *exchange*, understanding, and communication between institution and the community must be forged and used. The competitive and reciprocal nature of sub-systems in society must be realized and rendered to the degree appropriate and useful for planning and clinical care purposes. It must be realized that medicine in the community must first prove itself benevolent. Although it is easy to understand in the cross-cultural setting that professionals and altruistic action may be viewed as suspect by the indigenous population, this phenomenon is often obscured at home. Medicine when functioning at the grass roots level, is essentially guilty until proven innocent. Medicine cannot assume a partnership in its goals with the community or patient — it must negotiate a shared perspective.

Clinical epidemiology and new comprehensive models for health care are needed. Without altering the existing data base and current health care models used by clinicians and decision makers, change will not occur. Research and education are therefore vital. Medical educators need to be enlisted to train students and do research in psychological and social aspects of medicine. Support for a cadre of such practitioners and teachers is top priority. In addition, an acceptance of this approach needs to be fostered at the training, professional planning, and lay levels. Through research, education, social discourse, and context appropriate *action* we have a chance to create appropriate medical care.

REFERENCES

Berman, P. A. 1978. Village Health Workers in Java: Paper Presented at Conference on Medicalization of Society and Patient Compliance, Rochester, New York.

Carlson, R. 1975. *The End of Medicine.* New York: Wiley-Interscience.

Davis, M. M. 1916. Quoted in The Organization of Medical Services. *Am. Legislation Rev.* 6:16-20.

de Vries, M. 1981. A Plan for Mental Health Care in Swaziland. Report to African Development Bank.

Evans-Pritchard, E. E. 1937. *Witchcraft, Oracles and Magic among the Azandi.* London: Oxford.

Ferguson, A. E. 1981. Commercial Pharmaceutical Medicine and Medicalization: A Case Study from El Salvador. *Culture Med. Psychiatry* 5:105-34.

Fox, R. 1977. The Medicalization and Demedicalization of American Society. In *Doing Better and Feeling Worse*, ed. J. Knowles. New York: Norton.

Green, E. C. 1980. Roles for African Traditional Healers in Mental Health Care. *Med. Anthropology*, Fall, pp. 149-533.

Harwood, A. 1977. *Rx. Spiritualists As Needed.* New York: John Wiley.

Illich, I. 1976. *Medical Nemesis: The Expropriation of Health.* New York: Pantheon.

Knowles, J., ed. 1977. *Doing Better and Feeling Worse.* New York: Norton.

Kunitz, S. 1974. Professionalism and Social Control in the Progressive Era: The Case of Flexner Report. *J. Soc. Problems* 22:16-27.

Lipkin, M., Jr., and Kupka, K. 1982. *Psychosocial Factors Affecting Health.* New York: Praeger.

Lipkin, M., Jr., and Lybrand, W. A. 1982. *Population Based Medicine.* New York: Praeger.

McCorkle, J. 1961. Chiropractic: A Deviant Theory of Disease and Treatment in Contemporary Western Culture. *Hum. Organization* 20:20-23.

Ngubani, H. 1977. *Body and Mind in Zulu Medicine.* New York: Academic Press.

Pellitier, K. R. 1979. *Holistic Medicine: From Stress to Optimum Health.* New York: Delacorte and Delta.

Reiff, P. 1966. *The Triumph of the Therapeutic.* New York: Harper & Row.

Richmond, J. 1981. Health Behavior and Public Policy. Harvard Medical School, December 15, 1981.

Sedgwick, P. 1973. Illness: Mental and Otherwise. *The Hastings Center Studies* 1(3):19-40.

Stevens, R. 1971. *American Medicine and Public Interest.* New Haven, Conn.: Yale University Press.

Szasz, T. 1961. *The Myth of Mental Illness.* New York: Delta.

Turner, V. 1968. *Drums of Affliction.* Oxford: Clarendon.

White, K. L., and Bullock, P. 1980. *Health of Populations.* New York: Rockefeller Foundation.

CONTRIBUTORS

Robert L. Berg, M.D.
Department of Preventive, Family, and Rehabilitation Medicine
University of Rochester

Iman Bijleveld, Ph.D.
Department of Anthropology
Royal Tropical Institute
Amsterdam

Theodore M. Brown, Ph.D.
Department of History
University of Rochester

Donald J. Ciaglia
Department of Preventive, Family, and Rehabilitation Medicine
University of Rochester

Marten W. de Vries, M.D.
Department of Psychiatry
Harvard University

Horacio Fabrega, Jr., M.D.
Departments of Anthropology and Psychiatry
University of Pittsburgh

Ayala Gabriel, Ph.D.
Department of Anthropology
University of Rochester

Dean Harper, Ph.D.
Departments of Sociology and Psychiatry
University of Rochester

John M. Janzen, Ph.D.
Department of Anthropology
University of Kansas

Arthur Kleinman, M.D., M.A.
Departments of Psychiatry and Anthropology
University of Washington

Gerri S. Lamb, R.N., M.S.
School of Nursing
University of Rochester

Louis Lasagna, M.D.
Department of Pharmacology
University of Rochester

Christopher Lasch, Ph.D.
Department of History
University of Rochester

Mack Lipkin, Jr., M.D.
Division of Health Sciences
Rockefeller Foundation

Jane McCusker, M.A., Ph.D.
School of Public Health
University of Massachusetts, Amherst

John-Henry Pfifferling, Ph.D.
Center for Well-being of Health Professionals
Chapel Hill, North Carolina

Fitz John Porter Poole, Ph.D.
Department of Anthropology
University of Rochester

Jonathan Quick, M.D.
Duke-Watts Family Practice Program
Duke University

284

Lola Romanucci-Ross, Ph.D.
Department of Community Medicine
University of California at San Diego

Walter H. Sangree, Ph.D.
Department of Anthropology
University of Rochester

Randolph B. Schiffer, M.D.
Departments of Psychiatry and Neurology
University of Rochester

Corlien M. Varkevisser, Ph.D.
Department of Anthropology
Royal Tropical Institute
Amsterdam

285

INDEX

Aggrandizement, 209, 216; consequences of, 217
Agnatic blood (*kunum khaim*), 60, 65
Aid Post Orderly, 172
Alanon, 158
Alateen, 158
Alcoholics Anonymous (AA), 16, 151, 152, 158, 161, 278
Alcoholism, among American physicians, 194
Allopathic medicine, 175
American Anthropological Association annual meeting (1967), 242
American Indian Movement, 163
American Medical Association, 214, 215
American medical profession, late nineteenth century, 213
American Public Health Association, 213
American voluntary health agencies (VHAs), 220
Anthropologists, view of disease-illness and medical care, 19-34
Antibiotics, administration of, 224-25
Antivert, 110
Arrhythmias, life-threatening, 267
Australian Baptist Missionary Society, clinic of, 84; Bimin-Kuskusmin avoidance of, 84-88

Australian Naval Base, hospital at, 172

Bacon, Francis, 101
Bacteriology, 214; "halo effect," 218
BaKongo (Zaire), 10, 155
Balfour Beatty, Ltd., 243
Banganga, 10
Bantu Africa, modern medicine in, 8-14; introduction of, 13
Bantu African medical system, 3-4; divination in, 10-11
Bates, D., 6, 7
Bateson, G., 47
Bayes' theorem, 148
Bazelon, D. L., 38
Becker, M., 186
Bennett, J., 30
Berg, R. L., 152
Bettelheim, B., 102
Biggs, Hermann, 216
Bijleveld, I., 207, 248, 277
Bimin-Kuskusmin: belief system of, 51, 52; birth among, 54-88; ethnographic introduction, 58
Biomedicine, 46; overstatement of critiques in, 47-48; technical language of, 31
Birth among Bimin-Kuskusmin, 54-88; clinic, and skepticism, 84-88; determination of sex ritual, 68;